Career Options in
General Practice

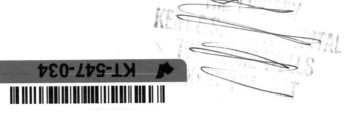

Edited by

Peter

Resear
Newho
Salarie

and

Petre

Gener
Traine
Newho

Forewo

Rhona

Radc
Oxfor

Radcliffe Publishing Ltd
18 Marcham Road
Abingdon
Oxon OX14 1AA
United Kingdom

www.radcliffe-oxford.com
Electronic catalogue and worldwide online ordering facility.

British Library Cataloguing in Publication Data

A catalogue record for this book is available from the British Library.

ISBN 1 85775 601 0

Typeset by Aarontype Ltd, Easton, Bristol
Printed and bound by TJ International Ltd, Padstow, Cornwall

Contents

Foreword   v
Preface   vii
About the editors   ix
List of contributors   x
Acknowledgements   xi

1   How hard do you want to work?   1
    Petre Jones

2   Partnerships   11
    Petre Jones

3   Salaried general practitioners   47
    Peter Aquino and Bhupinder Kohli

4   Locums   55
    Lise Hertel

5   Academic general practice   63
Sally Hull and Peter Aquino

6   Postgraduate education   71
Petre Jones

7   Is writing right for you?   81
Ruth Chambers

8   Working for a primary care trust   89
Peter Aquino, Bhupinder Kohli and Claire Davidson

9   Flexible working in general practice   97
Petre Jones and Farzana Hussain

10   Assorted hobbies   109
Petre Jones

Final thoughts   119
Index   121

Foreword

It is six years since I worked as a general practitioner but if there were the options then that there are now, my own career path would probably have been very different. Instead of being a full-time medical editor/journalist, I might still be working in a general practice in Glasgow but have the time and energy to do medical journalism on the side.

Even over the last six years, general practice has changed dramatically. Imagine being able to ask yourself the question, 'How hard do I want to work?' and fit your work around your life and other interests. General practice has become unique in this aspect. In my experience, young doctors have a much healthier attitude towards work/life balance than previous generations. They want to make general practice work for them rather than the other way around.

But, as a close friend (who works six sessions a week, pursues other interests and has just come back from a month's trekking holiday in the Himalayas) confided in me recently, 'This is great for me but I can see that if every GP works in a similar way, there will be no one to look after the patients. Someone must be getting dumped on!' However, I would caution you not to have such unselfish thoughts while reading this book. Instead, consider what would work for you, your personality, your family life and your interests.

Peter Aquino and Petre Jones previously wrote some articles for *Career Focus* to introduce our readers to general practice and the options available to them. The positive feedback I received from readers highlighted how helpful and useful their articles were. So, I am delighted that, along with some guest authors, they have spent the time and energy writing a book that discusses the current context of general practice and each training and working option in much more detail.

The in-depth discussion of advantages and disadvantages is particularly insightful and a useful decision aid. For example, if you detest paperwork then working as a salaried GP might be a feasible option for you but could you cope with the uncertainty over sick pay and the perception by some that you are a lower class of general practitioner? But this book is not just for those at the beginning of their career in general practice — more experienced GPs may be encouraged to rejuvenate their careers by taking up new hobbies and interests. How about becoming a GP trainer, writing for a newspaper, studying for a diploma or trying out sports medicine?

In my opinion, the authors have successfully produced an informed career guide with case histories, different perspectives and advice, in addition to important information. So delve in. I am sure that you will find what you are looking for.

Dr Rhona MacDonald MPCGP, MPH, DCH, DRCOG
Editor *Career Focus*, BMJ Careers
Senior editor of the Student *BMJ*
May 2004

Preface

General practice has always been a diverse specialty. Each practice is unique in its make up, the population it serves and the services provided, and the interests and personalities of the doctors. Even in Newham, the small area of East London where we both work, all the practices are different, and even the nine training practices offer different things to their registrars. Add to that all the extra little interests and roles that GPs can undertake, from occupational health work to drug abuse work, and you begin to see how wide the variety is in general practice.

Things are not getting simpler. With Government trying to bring more work into primary care, the creation of the GP with a special interest and the newer salaried posts, with or without special sessions, one can see why the newly qualifying GP might feel rather bewildered by the sheer choice facing them. They could become involved in academia, education, writing, secondary care work, outside agency work, or deepen their skills in general practice. Some will want to be partners, some salaried and some will want to work flexible hours because they have a life to lead outside general practice.

How do you negotiate these many choices? We hope that this book will be a useful guide to much of what is out there, and help training and newly qualifying GPs decide in what direction they want to head on the wide sea of their careers.

Of course it is not all about new GPs. Many of us who have been in general practice for a few years are looking for new challenges. Maybe life events have changed what is possible, or after 10 years doing the same thing it is time for something new. Certainly my life (*PJ*) has taken on a new direction since I left my old practice and started a new one in search of more flexibility, in my case due to illness. This book will provide some ideas for GPs looking for fresh direction within the profession, whether that is the challenge of BASICS (British Association of Immediate Care Doctors) work, the more measured world of benefits agency medicals or the fascination of professional education.

Medical students, who still get pitifully little exposure to general practice, will be interested to see some of the breadth and depth of what we do, and non-GPs, both in the profession in other specialties and those in management and politics, might even get some idea of what our specialty is about.

In writing this book we have revised and updated material from a series of articles in *BMJ Career Focus* and from the book *Partnerships in Practice* (Jones P (1999) *Partnerships in Practice: a GP's guide to getting it right first time*. Radcliffe Medical Press, Oxford), as well as adding a lot of new material, written by people who have experience of different types of general practice. As far as possible the authors are telling their stories warts and all from the inside. Sometimes we are biased; sometimes we are brutally honest. We hope you will agree in reading the book that the authors convey their interest and enjoyment in what they do. We are a group of quite different people who have found challenge and pleasure in our chosen careers at different points on the wide horizon that is general practice.

Peter Aquino
Petre Jones
May 2004

About the editors

Peter Aquino qualified as a doctor in 1994 and as a general practitioner in 2001. He has also undertaken further training in epidemiology and statistics and currently works as a research fellow in primary care epidemiology for Newham Primary Care Trust, East London.

Petre Jones qualified at Sheffield in 1985 and trained for general practice in East London, where he still works as a partner in a small practice and as a trainer and course organiser for the Newham vocational training scheme (VTS). His career, which has been influenced by recurrent illness, has included chairing a large training practice, running a small branch surgery, doing locums, working for a primary care organisation (PCO), bits of research, some writing and lots of teaching. His special interest is general practice, the encounter with the patient and the process of learning more about it.

List of contributors

Ruth Chambers
Professor of Primary Care Development, Staffordshire University
General Practitioner, Staffordshire

Claire Davidson
Clinical Lead in Diabetes, Newham Primary Care Trust
General Practitioner, Newham

Lise Hertel
General Practitioner, Newham

Sally Hull
Senior Lecturer, Department of General Practice and Primary Care,
Queen Mary and Westfield College
General Practitioner, Tower Hamlets

Farzana Hussain
General Practitioner Partner, Newham

Bhupinder Kohli
General Practitioner Partner, Newham

Acknowledgements

We would like to thank Rhona MacDonald, editor of *Career Focus* for the BMJ, for permission to use the material in Chapters 3 and 8, which originally appeared in *Career Focus*.

1

How hard do you want to work?

Petre Jones

Most of this book is about career choices in primary care and how to make the most of those opportunities. However, before we look at the jobs, this short chapter is about you, and what might suit you. We all have different backgrounds and circumstances, which affect the way we are able or want to work, and we all need to think about how to balance our work with the rest of our lives. For some, heavy financial commitments may mean that having a high income is paramount, whereas for others, family, illness and other interests may mean that shorter hours are important. There are no rules about what is right for you, only a whole set of choices to make − read on.

Welfare, workload and wad, the eternal triangle

Being happy with your job usually boils down to how you balance your workload and quality of patient care with the need to earn money and to remain healthy yourself. There is a common mind set in medicine which says that there is a difference between doctors and patients, and that doctors must always do everything they can for their patients, in an altruistic form of self-giving, and finally that it is not done to talk about money. So let me set the record straight.

Welfare

All of us at some point in our lives are patients. Whether we need simple contraception, help with an emergency, or help in dealing with long-term and life-threatening illness, ill health is part of what it is to be human, and so it will happen to you. Unfortunately many of us don't manage this very well. We self-medicate, deny our problems, ignore common referral pathways in favour of a 30-second chat with a mate in the corridor, and sometimes literally work till we drop. I suffer from a recurrent depressive disorder and have done all these and more. Even when we realise we have problems it is not that easy. It is hard for the doctor who has a doctor as a patient to deal with internal thoughts such as 'Am I doing this right?', 'What are they thinking of me?' (as if this were a clinical exam), and perhaps the most difficult, 'If *she* can be ill like this, it could really happen to me'. It is hard for the doctor patient too, often feeling a loss of power and vulnerable, and yet wanting to do things 'right'. She may alter her presentation of the illness 'to make it clearer for their colleague' and prepackage symptoms into classic syndromes. She may hide personal bits or just ignore important details. Finally, accessing appropriate treatment can be a nightmare. This is all material for another book, but there are two important points to make in relation to career choices.

Firstly, make sure you take out income protection insurance to an adequate degree when you are young, fit and think you do not need it. Too many colleagues have ignored this advice, have later become ill and then of course found themselves uninsurable and therefore, if ill again, may have no income at all. Of all the advice in this book I would count this as the most important .

Secondly, we need as a profession to develop a culture that recognises our humanity, and that means building flexibilities into jobs to support each other. In The Project Surgery in East London we have deliberately set out to do this.

- We are a small team of seven, working in small premises, and do not intend to expand. This is the sort of group size that can function supportively (consider the size of a well-functioning Balint group – about eight).
- We spend time together over lunch, with the whole team, and in the evenings about once every month, being ordinary people together.
- We try to manage working hours around childcare and healthcare parameters. For example, my work is fitted around psychotherapy sessions.
- Being able to be supportive to team members is written into person specifications.
- One partner brings her baby and au pair into the surgery so she can feel more comfortable because her baby is close by.
- We have a £20k contingency fund, built out of profits. This is to be used, for example, to cover locum costs if one partner needs rapid admission for healthcare.

The point of all this is that we are potentially vulnerable and the harder your workload, the higher your risk. Take care with how you structure your work and for many this will mean reducing income and also compromising somewhat on the desire to be the perfect general practitioner (GP). 'Good enough' is good enough. Think carefully about part-time work and flexibilities in working. Thankfully, the idea that you can work all day, all night and the next day and be okay is beginning to slip away from most areas of primary care. However, it will probably be some time before a culture of full support such as we are developing at The Project Surgery becomes commonplace.

Patient care

Patient care is clearly at the heart of what we do, and no one sets out to be Dr Dreadful. However, getting it right all the time is not possible. So, we have clinical governance frameworks that try to help us to get better most of the time, and this brings with it the extra workload of measuring stuff, learning more stuff and pushing ourselves to do better. At the extreme we find GPs happy to visit on request, do childhood immunisations at home and, even in this age of opt-outs and well-developed co-operatives, do all their own on-calls themselves. I am sure their patients love them, but this does bring a very heavy workload and this will have an impact on health and well-being. You might on the other hand consider the concept of being the 'good enough' GP to paraphrase Donald Winnicott's concept describing the equilibrium new parents hopefully reach after the fantasy of being the perfect parent, and the bad parent, both of which give rise to distress in parents.[1] GPs do not have to be perfect and can reasonably prioritise the more important aspects of care and put other stuff on the back burner without 'failing' their patients.

Money

Money is also important and it is generally true to say that in broad terms more work and more money tend to go together (although this does not explain why inner city GPs tend to earn less than leafy suburban GPs). There are issues about what money means to you in terms of self-image and perceived status. For some, and this is not really unreasonable, having a Mercedes is an important mark of having 'made it'. Unfortunately, they do not come cheap and this may involve working harder to achieve it. On the other hand, even the humblest lifestyle requires funding, and there are issues like housing, which have an influence on how much you need to earn. In London, for example, if a GP aspired to the same lifestyle as me, with a four-bedroom house in London, a Skoda car and not much else extravagant, they would need to earn about £20k per year more than me, just to cover the extra interest payments on the house because I bought it at the depth of the 1980s housing crash, and it has tripled in value since. So, think carefully about money. The problem with looking to increase income is that it will probably mean more work, which may affect your sanity, and more work may also mean cutting back on the quality of patient care.

The balance

The basic issue then for all doctors is to balance high quality patient care with income and your own sanity (Figure 1.1). If this seems to be overdramatic, consider what happens if people get the balance wrong. Too many partnerships break up over the issue of perceived workload — 'He doesn't actually give the clinical workload the same degree of priority that I do'. Feeling that patient care is being compromised in a bid to earn more money causes tension and partnership breakdown, and finally we hear with sad regularity of GPs ending their own lives because of perceived stress of the job.

The balance is set something like this. Generally the higher the list size the greater the income, but also the higher the list size the greater the workload; the higher the workload the greater the pressure to restrict patient care. Your personal position on these axes is more important than negotiating particular workloads. The workaholic will always overdo their work time, whatever is agreed, and the bone idle will always tend to dodge their responsibilities. However, a partnership of relaxed people in touch with their social side may get on well, and a partnership of keen innovators dedicated to patient care may also work. Join the wrong sort of partnership though and it will be a disaster.

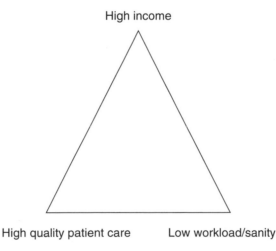

Figure 1.1   Workload is a balance between high income, quality patient care and one's own sanity.

Example 1
Doctor A decided not to join the five-doctor practice. It was clear that his perfectionism set him a high workload, which he could tolerate. Probably in any setting he would be a workaholic. The others had different priorities and values and set themselves different workloads. All would be successful doctors but they would not form a successful partnership.

Example 2
Doctor N joined his new practice realising that the workload would be high, although the financial rewards would also be high. He was used to a high workload, having worked for two years in a very busy obstetrics and gynaecology department before turning to general practice, and he enjoyed a challenge. He therefore coped well in his new practice.

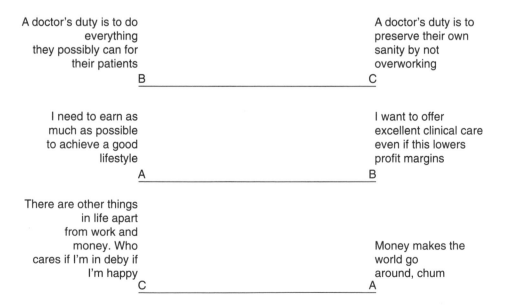

| A doctor's duty is to do everything they possibly can for their patients | | A doctor's duty is to preserve their own sanity by not overworking |
| B | | C |

| I need to earn as much as possible to achieve a good lifestyle | | I want to offer excellent clinical care even if this lowers profit margins |
| A | | B |

| There are other things in life apart from work and money. Who cares if I'm in deby if I'm happy | | Money makes the world go around, chum |
| C | | A |

Figure 1.2   Balancing income, workload and the quality of care.

Doing the triangle

Look at Figure 1.2 opposite. These are known as non-judgemental value rating scales (NJVRS), first developed by Roger Neighbour in his book *The Inner Apprentice*.[2] Each consists of a linear analog scale (pompous word for 'a line') set between two statements.

The statements are aimed to be the two ends of a spectrum of opinion, and you should mark off where you feel you would stand on each axis. You can then transfer your marks onto the sides of the workload triangle (Figure 1.3), being careful to keep each mark on the side in exactly the position as on the analog scale. So, if you

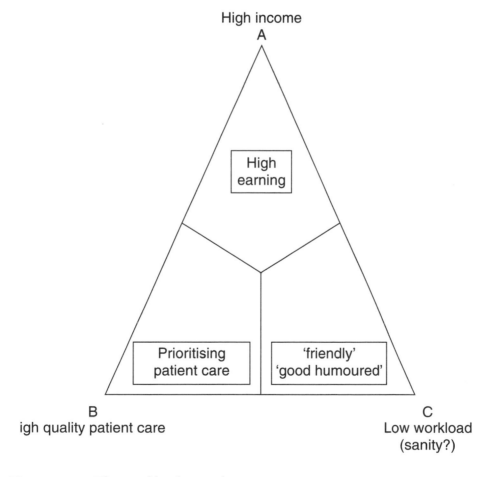

Figure 1.3   The workload triangle.

marked near to A on the AB axis, you will make sure you transfer it to near A on the AB side. Finally if you draw a line from each mark, to the opposite corner of the triangle, you will make another small triangle, inside the larger one (Figure 1.4).

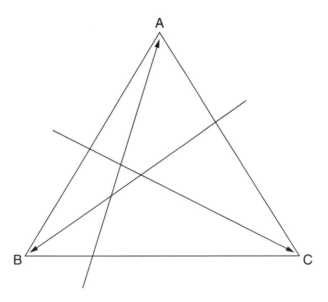

Figure 1.4   Example of a workload triangle.

Where the inner triangle falls gives you some idea of the choices you tend to make on the workload triangle. (Figure 1.4 is an example of a workload triangle for someone whose main priority is patient care at the expense of low workload/sanity.) If this feels comfortable then that is good, but if it feels uncomfortable for you, you might want to reflect on what it means for you. This is not meant to be a definitive personality test, but I have used this test with many groups and individuals over the last four years and it does seem to be fairly consistent and reliable in giving a view on people's core choices. This may help make it clearer to you how you want your career to go. When looking to join a partnership you might want to get all the partners to do the triangle. This might show something about what the practice believes, and would certainly be a con-versation starter.

References

1   Winnicott DW (1958) *Collected Papers: Through paediatrics to psychoanalysis.* Tavistock Publications, London; Basic Books, New York (1958); Hogarth Press and the Institute of Psychoanalysis, London (1975); Institute of Psychoanalysis and Karnac Books (1992); Brunner/Mazel, London (1992).
2   Neighbour R (1992) *The Inner Apprentice.* Kluwer, Lancaster.

2

Partnerships

Petre Jones

Partnership is still by far the commonest general practitioner (GP) working arrangement. Partnerships can be enormously supportive stable environments to provide GP care for patients, especially when the partners share common core values and working culture. However, nothing lasts for ever and, increasingly, people are feeling able to move from one partnership to another, perhaps not with ease, but not always with a re-enactment of the Somme either. In reality, like most human relationships, partnerships are usually 'good enough', with high and low points, but usually fit enough for the purpose, and the purpose is to enable you to provide a good service to your patients whilst generating enough profit for you to feel suitably rewarded for your pains. Some of us might want to add emotional support and friendship to the list, but a practice may function fine without this 'touchy-feely' stuff.

A partnership needs to function on three different levels and all are important in their different ways. Firstly there is the partnership deed. This is a major legal document that all partners have to agree to that sets out the legal terms and conditions under which the partnership will exist. Most deeds are fairly similar so I have tried to sketch out some of the important issues. A book like this cannot cover such a topic properly, and anyone thinking of signing, negotiating or changing a deed needs to get in touch with a solicitor, preferably one of the firms of specialist medical solicitors. The deed is the nearest thing to a contract that a partner has, and no one would think of taking a job without a contract. Strangely enough, some practices still do not have valid deeds. Every time a partner joins or leaves a partnership the deed needs to be updated or it becomes invalid, and some practices still do not have a deed at all. In these cases a partnership still exists called a 'partnership at will', governed by the Partnership Act of 1890. This is a strange piece of Victorian legislation that says, amongst other things, that any partner can dissolve the whole practice at any time just by saying so, and can then demand that all the assets of the partnership are sold and shared equally between the partners. Practice meltdown can then ensue. So, get a good partnership deed.

The second level on which a partnership has to function is to do with practice policies, and the fine detail of how the partnership will run the practice. Policies will cover issues such as who takes what management role, and therefore what type of practice manager you will need. How you feel about outside and specialty working, out-of-hours care, and how you try to distribute workload fairly are important issues. There are no rules on how to run a practice, only a series of choices to make in conjunction with your partners, and this is where partnerships start to take on their distinctive flavours. It is this variation, combined with the need to negotiate what you want, which makes the search for a partnership that is right for your needs challenging or, if you prefer, extremely intimidating and scary. So, it is worth taking time to think about exactly what you want (need) before looking for jobs. I have used some non-judgemental value rating scales (NJVRS), first designed by Roger Neighbour, to help you look at what choices you want to make.[1]

The final level to think about is the working culture of the practice. This is a mix of the personalities in the partnership, their individual backgrounds and the shared story and critical events that have coloured the way people relate to each other. This is the feel of the practice, the ethos, and has as much to do with the psychopathologies of the partners as it does to concepts of fairness and working priorities.

Partners' behaviour can sometimes be described more formally and labelled by psychologists, and this may give some extra insight into how the partnership works. It is easy to see how this would be important if you are going to work in a partnership for many years.

Box 2.1: Summary of key issues in partnerships

Deed level functioning
- Assessment and parity, shares and sale of good will.
- Leave.
- Premises.
- Outside work and particular interests.

Policies and working practices level functioning
- Management structure within the partnership.
- What type of manager?
- The status of salarieds and part-timers and hierarchy.

Practice 'feel' — support, formality, business-like, 'cuddly', etc.
- Team role.
- Conflict resolution styles.
- Partnership culture.

All of these levels of how partnerships work are important so I have tried to look at all of them in a bit more detail.

Culture and ethos

Key moral and professional stances

These are the issues that give a practice its character, and are expressions of the core beliefs of the practice. We all have core values although we may not think of them as such, and it is these which make us choose to work very hard or to be laid back, to fight for justice or to grab for ourselves, to yearn for novelty and truth or to stick with the familiar. Values such as this may not be easy to identify, but when the partnership is faced with choices, or put under stress (i.e. the everyday life of a practice), they will inform how partners think and behave. If your own core values are out of line with the rest of the practice you will feel uncomfortable, and when the chips are down you are likely to want to make different choices from your partners, resulting in principled disagreement. On the other hand, if all of the partners have identical core values you are likely to become a pretty stereotyped and lopsided practice. Some creative tension is good, to keep debate alive and avoid 'groupthink', a state of cosy collusion where no one dares to challenge the party line.

Example 1

Doctor A was approached by a five-doctor partnership to explore the possibility of becoming the sixth partner. They all knew each other very well professionally and Doctor A often did locum work for the partners, with which they were very impressed. They practised medicine in similar ways and all got on well with each other. However, Doctor A had a core value that he should always try to do the best possible job, otherwise he was letting himself down. The other partners felt that having personal boundaries was important, and so set limits on their working. The workaholic doctor A felt angry that the other partners' 'laziness' would diminish his work (and therefore self-worth) and the partners saw his perfectionism as a threat to their self-defences. Doctor A did not join the partnership.

Example 2

Three doctors of different ages and medical styles, from different cultural and ethnic backgrounds, all shared the same core value about the immense worth of individual patients, and a shared sense of spirituality, albeit expressed in three different religious traditions. They formed a very strong partnership.

Example 3

With three children at private school and a big mortgage on his home and surgery building, Doctor B needed money! He was hardworking and independent and greatly valued his family's comfortable lifestyle, which to him was a mark of success. He could not afford to risk a partner not working as hard as he did, so although he had a series of assistants, he never looked for a partner.

The stereotypes and self-labelled identity – the practice culture

The core values of the practice, together with its collective experience and corporate stories, lead to a practice's identity. Obviously there is a whole spectrum of types and styles of practice but some stereotypes can be identified, and often practices will label themselves as 'friendly' or 'academic' for example.

More seriously, many practices have carefully thought through moral, political or religious stances with which they identify themselves. Consider what type of practice might suit your core values. Do you want to be in a co-operative practice where each person, from cleaner to partner, earns the same and shares decision making? Are all partners paid-up members of the Medical Practitioners' Union (MPU) taking a solid socialist stand? Does the practice take a particular moral stand for example on termination of pregnancy? Would you describe yourself as a 'Christian practice', or for that matter a 'Jewish practice' or is this something you would be looking for? I have not seen 'Muslim practice' or any other religious description given to a practice yet, although I have known practices informally describing themselves with an ethnic label! Where does legitimate unique identity end and cliquish 'groupthink' begin?

Groupthink is a state that any close-knit group of people can get into where their desire to stick together, and not rock the boat, overrides their motivation to think clearly and objectively. The group is seen as invulnerable and never wrong, and outsiders are seen with a degree of suspicion. It will be hard to express a view that goes against the party line and so there is an illusion of unanimity. Unfortunately this leads to a lack of debate and a reluctance to seek outside advice. If a practice ends up like this it can be painful to break out, but the danger of groupthink is that it leads to significant underperformance and therefore poorer patient care.

In many practices the ethos is not labelled as such, being more an unspoken framework of norms within which members operate, without ever being put into words. The practice may be friendly, caring and hardworking, or disorganised, stressed, paranoid and grumpy, respecting the rights of professionals and patients, or self-centred with everyone for themselves. There is also an important balance to be struck between, on the one hand, conflicting values leading to unhelpful confrontation and even open warfare and, on the other, cliquish collusion which, ostrich-like, ignores challenges and rational debate. You can only find all this out by talking to people, spending time in the practice and keeping your antennae out.

In the end all practices are a mixture of good and bad elements so there is no perfect set up, but in the end the partnership culture is the thing that will have more influence on your happiness and wellbeing at work than any other, so take care to explore this.

The partnership dynamic and partners' behaviour

The way partners relate to each other in both formal and informal settings (e.g. in partners' meetings and over lunch) is vital to a practice, but may be very hard to pin down or put into clear thoughts. The key question is, 'Can this group of individuals find a way to comfortably work together and respect each other?'

Issues like joining a husband and wife who are partners, or partnerships with open conflict between partners, are situations which one would have to be very careful with, although both can actually work. Talk to partners and ex-partners and anyone else who may be in the know to find out as much as possible about internal politics and personalities. In the end gut feeling may be the best guide.

Team roles

Are you good in a team, and why? What are your strengths and weaknesses? Are you a solitary worker, or a collaborator? Are you something of an independent free thinker (others may say a loose cannon), or do you like to have clear rules laid down and work to guidelines and protocols? What role do you tend to play in a team —

chair, plant, monitor/evaluator, team player? Obviously it is desirable to have an eclectic mix within the team; it is chaos if everyone is an independent free thinker, but fossilised if no one ever challenges the status quo!

Some practices do psychological profiling of prospective new partners to see if they are likely to fit into their team, often by using questionnaires, but most are not quite that organised (or obsessional).

Work by Belbin on management teams in industry has shown that the best functioning management teams have a chair and a plant and a mix of others.[2] So it seems that it is good to have someone who has the courage and insight to stir things up a bit and someone else

---

Box 2.2: Belbin's group roles

Consider which of these best describes you at work:

- company worker   conservative, dutiful, predictable
- chair   calm, self-confident, controlled
- shaper   highly strung, outgoing, dynamic
- plant   individualistic, serious minded, unorthodox
- resource investigator   extrovert, enthusiastic, curious, communicative
- monitor/evaluator   sober, unemotional, prudent
- team player   socially orientated, mild, sensitive
- completer-finisher   painstaking, orderly, conscientious, anxious.

These terms refer to how people tend to function within a team, and are not personality types, although they may be related to personality. A person with an obsessional personality might function in a particular team as a monitor/evaluator, or as a completer-finisher, or as a company worker, or as a chair, depending on what other roles were being played, so it is possible to adapt to the needs of a team. However, each person will be most comfortable with a particular role, so a team of natural plants is just not likely to work.

with the calm strength to hold it all together and bring things to a negotiated conclusion. All the different roles are useful in different ways (Box 2.2).

Conflict resolution styles

Another way of looking at how people function in groups is to look at how they deal with disagreement and conflict. Some people are naturally spiky and fight their own corner hard, without bothering too much about how others feel, whilst at the other end of the spectrum others are so keen to make things seem okay for everyone else they sacrifice their own voice and never feel able to express their own needs and thoughts for fear of upsetting people.

Thomas and Kilmann, in their Conflict Mode Instrument, describe five styles that people fall into in terms of their ways of dealing with conflict.[3] Based on a person's assertiveness and concern for other people's needs, they characterised the styles by comparing them to animals (Table 2.1).

It is probably best to have a mixture of styles within a team, but certainly at least one owl (who might also be the Belbin shaper). It is a good idea to think about which style you tend to use, and look at the ways other partners behave in any practice you look at. If conflict is never faced up to, because everyone is a teddy bear or a tortoise, simmering resentments and silent collusions will eventually undermine relationships. However, if there is a team of sharks, only the 'strongest' will survive.

Number of partners

Obviously this is key to how a practice works, but for equally obvious practical reasons there is limited room for manoeuvre on this. You will wish to consider these issues when looking round at prospective practices.

Larger practices

In an inner city area like Newham, a large practice might have four to six partners, although in national terms this is really medium-sized.

Table 2.1   Conflict mode styles and their characteristics

Style	Priorities	Description	Comment
Tortoise	Assertiveness low Others' needs low	Avoids conflict and retreats into shell, giving up personal goals and others' needs	Helpless
Teddy bear	Assertiveness low Others' needs high	Always wants to make things okay for other people, disregarding own needs (or under-valuing self)	Nice to have around until the issues get tough
Fox	Assertiveness mid Others' needs mid	Will tend to look for middle ground and compromise to end conflict	Engages with disagreement but tends to sacrifice own and others' needs
Owl	Assertiveness high Others' needs high	Will stick with a conflict situation and work towards a win/win resolution	Strong person in a team, but perhaps rather intense
Shark	Assertiveness high Others' needs low	Fights own corner hard to get what they want, sometimes trampling on toes	If your needs coincide with theirs, good; if not, beware

There are a number of advantages to this size of practice (this is my bias coming out again – ours is a four-partner practice). Sharing of skills and resources within a team allows a wide range of services to be provided and responsibility for running the practice can be shared. There is therefore more scope for teamwork, sharing of stress and efficiency. A larger practice will tend to have more influence at PCO and health authority level than an individual small practice and may therefore be in a stronger position to fight for resources or set local priorities, unless a small practice makes this sort of work a major practice activity.

On the other hand, the larger the number of partners the greater the potential for disagreement over core values, money or clinical work. To overcome this, there will need to be an investment of time to make partnership relationships work, and more formal boundaries set to guide how partners interact. As a result, meetings may have to be more formal and management structures more clearly defined, making large practices seem less personal, at least at first.

There is a trend nationally, although not yet seen in the inner cities, towards the 'superpractice' of 12 or more (occasionally many more) partners in the same practice. As we work more closely together in primary care trusts (PCTs) and co-operatives this trend may grow, turning the practice from being a small or medium-sized business into a sizeable corporation. My own view on this was summarised once by a friend of mine who, as a patient, had moved to a town in which there were only two practices, each with 12 doctors. She commented, like someone feeling the passing of their youth, 'You can't have your own doctor any more'. I would be sad to see personal and continuous care disappear.

Small practices linked

Some smaller practices prefer to work in a linked but arms-length relationship. They may share premises, cover each other for on-call work, or share resources or practice staff. At the same time they remain separate practices with their own financial and management processes. This is very likely to be a way forward for inner city areas where small practices are increasingly working together. Obviously it is up to each practice to decide which areas they wish to collaborate on and which they wish to remain separate on, and the terms on which they will work.

The main advantage of this approach is that you can remain 'just good friends' rather than being 'married', so there is more freedom and flexibility. This may be particularly appropriate for some local circumstances, for example where premises pose limitations, or rural geography limits the closeness with which doctors can sensibly work.

However, there are some drawbacks. There will be significant duplication of resources, particularly administratively (e.g. do you each employ a practice manager or club together to share perhaps a more skilled manager?). There will also be less support within each practice and a narrower range of services will be available than in one larger practice.

If practices choose to work in this way it is worth asking why. Why do they want to work together at all; what can't they do on their own? On the other hand, why haven't they formed a full partnership? It might be that a group of people who really do not get on well have been thrown together by circumstances but feel unable to form a partnership relationship. Perhaps linking smaller practices is a pragmatic half-way house that is without a firm foundation and therefore inherently unstable.

Example 4

In the 'Golden Age' of general practice before the 1990 imposed contract there was a Red Book payment called the group practice allowance, to encourage single-handed doctors to work more closely together. So it was that four doctors working independently in the same health centre decided to form loose links. They decided to share a practice manager and administrative staff, but remain independent doctors. This worked for a while but because the doctors continued to work and think as individuals it became very hard for them to agree, and they soon spent most of the time arguing. They had not got enough investment in joint working. They returned to being single-handed practices after the rather weak glue of the group practice allowance was abolished.

Example 5

As a quirk of history two practices with two partners each grew up close to each other. Each had a spare room in their premises. One converted their spare room into a treatment room, whilst the other converted theirs into a counselling room. By an arrangement of sharing premises and jointly employing a sessional counsellor they were then both able to offer minor surgery and counselling services to their patients. It is easy to see this arrangement developing closer links between the practices, in a European Union (EU) style 'ever closer union'.

Small practices

Single-handed practice is not really what this chapter is about but it has its own attractions as a flexible and independent way of working, and will remain a significant part of the general practice picture, particularly in inner city areas. However, two- and to some extent three-handed practices have their own unique partnership issues. With nowhere to hide and no one to mediate, the practice hinges critically on the nature of the relationship between the partners. If they can work openly and honestly together then things will go well, but if there is significant disagreement then divorce is all too common. For example, within Newham, an area with a high proportion of single-handed practices, many of these have arisen out of partnership disputes within two- and three-handed practices. On the other hand there are examples where a small partnership is strong.

Example 6
Doctor C joined a practice with three other doctors, D, E and F. Unknown to her, D and E were finding it hard to get on with F, who had joined the practice only 10 months earlier. C ignored her gut feelings of unease but soon after joining it became clear that she was also having problems relating to F and was tending to side with D and E. Eventually, after much heartache on both sides, F, who was struggling with marriage problems which he had tried to hide from the practice, moved on to another practice and C, D and E continued as a partnership. All those involved were haunted by the difficulties for several years.

Example 7
Doctor G was invited to become a partner in the practice in which she had been a registrar. The four existing partners were robust with each other and partners' meetings tended to end in votes with a predictable two/two split. In effect there were two opposing parties within the partnership. Doctor G was

well aware of this when she agreed to join. She was a non-confrontational but strong character who enjoyed having the balance of power. She quickly took the role of chair and the whole partnership dynamic softened.

Policies that shape a practice

Some more formal models of how the practice runs and partnership dynamics can be pinned down fairly easily and give clues to the less formal aspects. This is the level of the formal practice policy.

Senior partner as executive

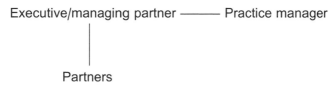

In this quite simple model, one partner, perhaps the 'senior' partner, leads on most decisions and chairs the partnership. He works quite closely with the practice manager, if there is one, and will delegate tasks to partners as necessary. This sounds autocratic but may work well with a sensitive executive who is a natural lead figure and has appropriate management skills. Obviously the other partners need to feel comfortable with a more subordinate role, but are freer to indulge other medical interests.

A key advantage of this model is that lines of decision making are clear within the practice which helps the practice manager, and it will be clear to those outside the practice, such as the health authority, who to relate to. This can put a lot of pressure though on the executive partner, who may well need a lower clinical load and extra time to do the management work.

On the negative side having one powerful figure within the partnership can lead to tension and resentments. At some point a young lion/old lion conflict is very likely, but then no single dynamic will last for ever. Practices evolve. However, this model limits the management skill and time of the practice to those of the executive, so that other partners may have no opportunity (or are not forced by circumstances) to develop these skills. What then happens when the executive is on holiday, or ill with his ulcer, or is convicted of fraud?

Democracy and shared responsibility

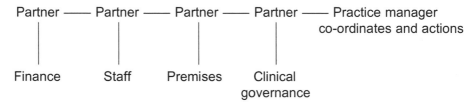

In this model the partners all work together and have equal power within the partnership, but divide up the responsibility for the key management functions between them. Each partner will make simple decisions in their own area of responsibility in conjunction with the practice manager, but for larger issues they will bring the matter to the partners' meeting for a full discussion. This is a sort of cabinet-style structure.

The advantages of this system are that it is fair to each partner and it respects each person's strengths. It is possible to match the tasks to partners' skills, for example making the monitor/evaluator responsible for clinical governance, or the obsessive with financial skill in charge of money. The management load is spread between all the partners and all are involved in some leadership, building trust within the practice, and capitalising on the breadth of skills available. Rapid response to change becomes possible with partners working autonomously in their own areas of responsibility with the practice manager.

There is no such thing as a free lunch. The down side of this system is that a large management team can lead to confusion. It may be difficult to deal with issues which cross boundaries of partners' responsibility, and there must be a high degree of trust between partners. To maintain this there will need to be a lot of discussion time, and a self-confident manager. Another disadvantage is that not all partners may wish to be heavily involved in running the practice.

Management team within a partnership

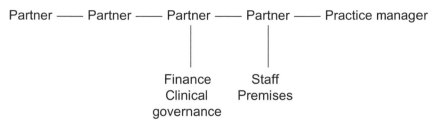

Partner —— Partner —— Partner —— Partner —— Practice manager

Finance
Clinical
governance

Staff
Premises

This is similar to the model described in the previous section, but with some partners choosing to stay out of managing the practice. This will be very flexible to partners' needs, but the back seat partners may feel marginalised and disempowered. Meanwhile, the managing partners may feel resentful about their extra work and responsibility, and working out how to balance giving the management team time to manage, lightening the clinical load for the managers and considering altering partnership shares to reflect the new workload regime is fraught with potentially partnership breaking issues.

Everyone makes decisions together

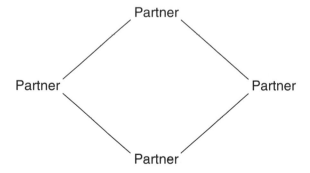

Partner

Partner

Partner

Partner

As the diagram suggests this can be a nice cosy way to do things. On the surface it sounds attractive. Everyone is consulted, and then you either act on the consensus of all the partners or the will of the majority, depending on how you want to work it. This may work for a very small practice, but in a medium or large practice it would take a long time to make decisions if all the partners had to agree everything, unless you are going to spend a lot of time in partners' meetings. If a large practice, or even a medium-sized practice, adopts this type of decision making it may suggest a problem. Perhaps the partners have not really thought about management issues and run the practice as a cottage industry rather than a modern business. Maybe they are lacking in trust for one another, or are unhappy taking the risk of making decisions on behalf of other people without discussing things with them. Of course you may feel that these so-called problems are in fact excellent qualities for doctors and could be called sensitivity to others, a respect for human scale values and focusing on people rather than processes. It is all a matter of how you view things.

Joint responsibility for decisions

Being in partnership means you share legal responsibilities. For example, you jointly employ staff and are therefore jointly responsible for employment law issues. You are also jointly liable for most practice debts. (Interestingly you are now not jointly liable for tax debts, only for your own share of the partnership tax.) So if one partner unfairly dismisses a staff member, the whole partnership can be taken to an industrial tribunal, or if one partner runs up a huge bill on the practice account, the partnership will still have to pay. So the critical question is do you trust your partners? Will you be happy to accept majority voting and majority decisions, even when you disagree?

How will formal decisions be made?

Whichever management model you adopt you will still need to agree a mechanism by which formal partnership decisions are made. One possibility is working by consensus, where all partners agree informally before decisions are taken, or you may prefer to formalise it with voting and do things only on a unanimous vote.

This would rapidly become unworkable in all but the smallest practices (try getting any group of GPs to all agree on anything!) and so, as with the ever-expanding EU, there will have to be some decision making by majority voting. (You might want to be a bit careful in a three-partner practice where two partners are married!) If you use a voting system, you will still need to work out which decisions will be decided by majority vote and which by unanimous vote. Major policy issues like a change in practice area would probably need to be unanimous and any change in the partnership deed, the partners' governing contract with each other, has to be unanimous. Smaller issues could be decided on a majority basis, but it can be hard to draw the line between major and smaller decisions. Perhaps the partnership deed should include some illustrative examples.

You might even want to consider a system of qualified majority voting where for example a two-thirds majority is needed to do something. It can get very complicated. Perhaps it would be wise to take some time to reflect on what each of these systems says about the dynamic of the partnership?

Example 8
A five-doctor practice used to work with an executive partner system and their partnership shares were weighted so that the executive partner drew a slightly larger share than the others. As the work of a modern practice built up the partners changed the way they worked to a shared responsibility system. Before long the four previously junior partners realised that the existing partnership shares were unjust with shared responsibility, but knew that to change shares would require unanimous agreement, which would not be easy to get! However, money was tight for two of them, and they felt that to keep the current shares could represent an illegal sale of good will (*see* section below). At a tense and frank partnership meeting they confronted the issue and with a unanimous decision they altered the shares to reflect true workload.

Example 9
In a three-partner practice, one partner was on long-term sick leave. On her return she found that the other two partners had made a decision to spend £2000 on a new autoclave, which she felt was not really needed. This was not, however, a major policy decision, and their partnership deed provided for simple majority voting for routine decisions, so she bit the bullet and paid her share.

Practice manager or practice administrator?

The person in charge of managing the practice organisation is pivotal, and influences both the work of the partners and the style and culture of the practice. No two practice managers seem to do quite the same job, but there are in fact two reasonably distinct species in this genus that are fairly easy to identify. Confusingly, both types are called practice manager. You may be happier with one or other type depending on how you wish to work, but if you employ the wrong type for your practice it could get very uncomfortable.

The first type could be called 'true managers'. These people will be proactive in making decisions and have a professional management approach, managing the practice and its various components (finance, staff, premises and equipment, time, systems, teams, etc.) rather than the practice being managed by the partners, and they will take a strong strategic role in the practice. They will obviously have strong management skills and training and will have sound assertiveness skills. They are expensive to employ, but are very good at encouraging innovation and change and, through this, practice and team development. A 'true manager' will take a lot of the administrative burden off the partners and may well be able to increase income. For example, by perfecting internal systems, such as the item-of-service claiming routine, you may find that maternity or contraceptive fee claims are increased, or the manager may well know ways of working the Red Book to your advantage. The details of the Red Book are esoteric and most doctors do not fully understand it (or have the time or motivation to learn about it), especially things like advance leave payments, dispensing regulations or the fee for arrest of a dental haemorrhage. A good 'true manager' will navigate the Red Book with some skill. This would of course help to offset the higher salary.

The second type of practice manager could be called 'practice administrators'. These professionals will run the administrative side of the practice and do (or delegate) the routine tasks like pay roll and keeping tabs on income and expenditure and Red Book payments. However, unlike 'true managers', 'administrators' would not be expected to take a strategic view of practice development or seek to 'manage' the partners. Rather, the partners would very much remain in control of the business, and not encourage the administrator to make proactive innovation. Although often very experienced, administrators are generally paid on a lower salary scale, and are more likely to be affordable by smaller practices. They are also less threatening to GPs who feel that the partners own the business and should therefore run it.

 If you want to be very much in control then an administrator may be right for you, particularly if you have strong management skills and time to spend on it. On the other hand, if you want to be an innovative practice but feel you lack management skills and experience you may prefer a true manager.

Example 10
A well-established practice with one principal and two assistants felt a need to innovate. They needed new premises and wanted to expand their team and the services they offered. They appointed a new and enthusiastic manager who had a lot of experience as a deputy practice manager in a practice in another village, and wanted to move his career on. After a few months it became clear that the principal had difficulty handing over control, making staff decisions without talking to the manager and not letting him in on discussions with the health authority about the new building. The manager felt he had less responsibility than in his previous job and so moved on to another job.

Example 11
A five-partner practice was struggling to keep up with its management work. They were an innovative training practice with a manager approaching retirement who worked as an 'administrator'. When she retired, a new manager, very much of the 'true manager' type, was appointed. She was able to rebuild the organisation and help progress practice development, and make a significant difference to the partners' stress levels.

Attitude to part-time or job share

Many of us like the idea of job share or part-time working, with its flexibility to fit around family, academic or other commitments and the potential for lower stress levels. It seems likely that this type of working will become more common in the future despite the lower earnings potential, but this will have an impact on practices.

More partners means more relationships within the partnership. This makes working relationships harder to negotiate, with more potential for disagreement, and there is a greater need for more formal frameworks within the practice. You might have to have a more formal committee structure for partnership meetings, or more structured ways of communicating with each other. However, having more people in the team increases the skills base, so you may be able to broaden your practice services. Part-timers often say they have less influence within the practice, and full-timers often perceive part-timers as having less commitment and not being able to take the pace.

'Salaried partners'

There is no such thing as a salaried partner. A partner is a self-employed person who owns a share of the business and draws a share of the profits, usually a percentage share, the exact value of which will vary with the profits. Someone drawing a fixed salary is an employee, with different tax liabilities and employment rights. A salaried person has rights to go to an industrial tribunal and sick leave rights, for example. They are also subject to the terms of a contract, to work certain set hours for example. A partner could, however, draw a fixed share (a fixed sum rather than a percentage) of the profit. He is then legally a partner, with the full rights of a partner, to see the accounts for example, and is a principal in general practice, but without some of the financial risks and benefits of being an ordinary percentage share partner. Having a fixed share might be an alternative to percentage share in the period leading up to parity because it would give you a clearly defined income without having to work out the vagaries of income streams and expenses.

Salaried GPs

True salaried GPs are not at all part of the partnership, of course, but the attitude of partners to them says something important about the practice. If salaried GPs are comfortably part of the practice educational and teamwork meetings, and all GPs are happy to chip in with clinical work, it suggests a sense of mutual respect for each others' role and a level of equality in working together. However, an alternative way of seeing things is for the partners to feel that as they run the practice they are more important than salaried GPs, and a hierarchy forms, with the senior partner at the top, then partners, then salarieds, then perhaps registrars. Hierarchy in administration staff, from practice manager down to junior receptionist, also commonly exists. Whether people are referred to in first name terms gives a pretty good clue to hierarchy. Neither approach is wrong, but you may feel more comfortable with one approach rather than the other and this is one area which is very difficult to change.

Patients and personal lists

How will you divide up the patients? Personal lists, where patients are restricted as far as possible to seeing their registered doctor, encourage continuity of care but are administratively difficult. What do you do in an emergency when the patient's doctor is away for example? It may be worth overcoming these problems if the partners work in very different ways, but it will be harder to develop and audit practice policy and protocols with doctors working quite separately. Do you want to deny patients the right to choose to see a different doctor for a particular problem? Personal lists also make it hard to develop areas of clinical interest within the practice. Minor surgery, for example, has to be done by a partner who is on the minor surgery list. Will a minor surgery partner do procedures on other partners' lists? If not, for the sake of personal lists you will reduce services and restrict income. If they will, the logic of personal lists starts to break down. There are many similar situations which make a rigid personal list system hard to maintain.

Issues for the partnership deed

The partnership deed is the key bedrock document for the partnership. It will be drawn up by a solicitor, preferably a specialist medical solicitor, and defines the formal relationship between the partners. It must be updated whenever there is a change in the partnership.

Joining and leaving the practice

Mutual assessment periods and progression to parity

All parties will be keen to establish firm secure working relationships as quickly as possible when a partner joins a practice, but will also be wary of making a firm commitment too soon. It is therefore wise to look at agreeing a mutual assessment period, of say six months, at the end of which time either side can walk away from the deal without rancour or blame. Sometimes partnerships, like relationships, do not always work out. This gives both sides a pressure-free period to see how things go, but how long should this be? Clearly this must be agreed. Like engagements, if the mutual assessment period is too short you risk making a big mistake (partnership splits are as traumatic as divorce, but more expensive), but if too long it sends a message of reluctance to make commitments, and a fear that the new person will be dumped. The new person will be a full legal partner during this time, on whatever share is agreed, but may have less power in the partnership.

Mutual assessment is not the same as progression to parity, which is the length of time it will take for the new partner to draw a share equal to everyone else from the pooled income (items like seniority payments are often retained by the partner they relate to and not put in the pool for sharing), and pro rata for part-timers. The progression to parity could start at the same time as a mutual assessment period or after the final commitment is made.

The justification for progression to parity is that a new partner will not take as much responsibility for running the practice as the existing partners. Exactly what share a new partner draws in the time to parity is a matter of negotiation, but no partner should draw less than one-third of the drawings of the highest earner (pro rata for part-timers). Some practices are happy to do away with progression to parity altogether, and at the other extreme, periods of greater than two to three years are suspect.

Compulsory expulsion

In the partnership deed there will be a clause about the circumstances in which you might be required to resign from the practice. These are worth thinking about. Many of these circumstances are obvious, for example if you are struck off the medical register, but there may be conditions where you might feel expulsion would be inappropriate or discriminatory. You will never imagine that these clauses might be used, but it is worth thinking a little about what might lead to expulsion. What is a hanging offence? Make sure there is a clause to cover the partnership if one partner does commit 'treason against the partnership', but also make sure that partners are not inadvertently exposed to unfair expulsion. There is, of course, no recourse to an industrial tribunal for unfair dismissal. You are self-employed.

Restrictive covenants on leaving

A restricted covenant clause is a section of a partnership deed that restricts what a partner who leaves can do after leaving. You might for example agree that a partner who leaves may not treat patients who are on the practice list at the time they leave for at least one year. This type of covenant may safeguard the practice if a partner leaves with his list of 2000 patients and sets up shop next door, but may be unfair to a new person who might want to leave if things go wrong but who still wants to work locally. If the covenant is too broad, for example you would not be permitted to see any patients living within five miles of the practice for five years in an urban area, then the whole covenant is void and unenforceable. In summary, restrictive covenants must be fair and reasonable to both sides.

Example 12
In a six-partner urban practice five partners got on well, but one partner, Doctor K, was isolated. He disagreed with the others on

many partnership issues, and staff found him hard to deal with. His presence seemed to paralyse the practice, but because he had not breached any part of the partnership deed he could not be required to leave.

Example 13
In a practice of four doctors, one partner, Doctor L, became un-expectedly ill with an acute severe depression. He had no past history but was admitted to hospital as an informal patient, although the severity of the illness would have warranted com-pulsory admission if he had refused to go. After a year Doctor L was able to return to work full-time. However, the partner-ship deed said that if a partner was compulsorily admitted under Section 2 or 3 of the Mental Health Act 1983 he could be ex-pelled from the partnership. There were other reasonable provi-sions for sick leave for physical or mental illness. At the time the deed was drawn up no one really looked at this clause: it would never happen to them. When Doctor L recovered it was felt that the clause discriminated against mental illness, and was struck out, much to the relief of Doctor L who continues to live with the knowledge that his depression could recur.

Leave

When it comes to leave arrangements you will need to balance the sanity and humanity of the partners against the cost of locums (or the increased workload for the other partners if you choose to go for an internal cover arrangement). You will need to either consider some sort of policy on locum employment to cover leave, or agree to cover each other's time off.

The following nine types of leave are dealt with in our partnership deed. You might wish to consider terms for any or all of these types of leave.

● *Annual leave*   Six weeks is common, but remember the cost. Will it be okay for more than one partner to be away at a time? Much will depend on the practice size.

- *Study leave*   You will need some study leave for continued professional development, but do you really want to cover your partner whilst he enjoys a three-week postgraduate education allowance (PGEA) course in Portugal, brushing up his golf? Do you want a say in what a partner takes study leave for?

- *Sick leave*   This is straightforward for short periods, but what about longer sick leave: will you need individual insurance to cover the costs of this? Will the sick partner have to pay locum costs, or will the practice, and for how long? If the health authority will not pay locum costs you will need to ensure that each partner has their own locum expenses policy.

- *Maternity leave*   You are self-employed so not covered by the usual employment rules although the maternity leave deal must not be worse than an equivalent sick leave deal for a male partner. It seems very strange to me that maternity leave should be compared to sick leave, but that is employment law. Make sure you build in a deal that is acceptable to you.

- *Paternity leave*   This is very trendy, and necessary believe me. I speak as a father of five. How long will you give a new dad? In one practice they allow four weeks, but this is an area in which attitudes are changing rapidly, so take a look at national rules for the employed before taking a decision. Remember, you may have completed your family but the newly married partner with strong views on contraception may take a special interest in this clause.

- *Sabbatical leave*   Leaving for three months or more can cause major practice disruption so how often do you want partners to go off for long periods, and who will fund it? Sabbaticals are very attractive to the partner taking them, who may see this as a way to revive a tired career, and come back refreshed.

- *Compassionate leave*   You cannot in all humanity make hard and fast rules about compassionate leave, but rough guides and examples in the deed may give you a framework on which to base 'on the hoof decisions' should the need ever arise.

- *Religious observance leave*   Will you make special provision for pious members of the practice to observe the major holy days of their tradition? Is this fair to the godless partners? You might consider having an agreement that partners should not be asked to be on call on a major holy day of their tradition other than in exceptional circumstances.

- *Adoption leave*   This is an equivalent to maternity leave or paternity leave which gives new adoptive parents the same rights as natural parents.

Owning or leasing the premises

This is a hugely complex issue, that can only really be touched on here, but is probably less important for new partners than you might think, which is surprising given the amount of money involved.

Own (and control) the premises

If the partners own the premises they will have control over them and be responsible for them.

In order to own a share of the property a partner would have to raise the capital, which could easily amount to anything up to £300k at 1999 prices. This is likely to come as a loan with interest payments, and when you compare this to your mortgage costs it sounds witheringly expensive. However, the interest payments should be covered by the cost rent or notional rent payments from the health authority to the practice for the privilege of using your privately owned building for NHS work, in seeing NHS patients. Interestingly, if you do too much private work in your building (in excess of 10% of practice income) the health authority will reduce their payments. With the interest thus taken care of, you only have to worry about the capital invested. You might choose to pay this off gradually so that when you retire you can sell your share of the building to the next partner, giving you a nice little lump sum. Alternatively, if this sort of investment is not for you, you could maintain the loan as a business debt, in which case you do not have to sink money into it but you will not get anything back on retirement, and you continue to have a massive debt until you have found someone to buy it from you.

When a partner leaves, their share can be bought by the other partners or their successor at the latest market rate and they will then get the rent payments. The leaving partner, on selling, will get back their original investment plus any growth due to building price inflation. You may also wish to put a clause in the partnership deed to say that the leaving partner does not have to sell their share for less than they paid for it, to avoid negative equity problems in the event of a property slump.

Thus taking out a loan for £300k can be seen as a pension investment which may be quite worthwhile, like getting the interest payments on your mortgage paid by the health authority whilst you stand to gain, effectively free of cost, any growth in the capital investment, with a guarantee that you will not lose.

However, with ownership of the building comes the responsibility for it, and the risk associated with a huge investment. Having a large financial commitment like this may tie a partner down, particularly at the start of their career as a principal, when they may feel they might wish to move practices at some point. New partners may also be justifiably nervous of the risk given the pace of change in the NHS. In some practices some of the partners own the building with their partners taking no role in it, depending on their personal feelings about financial risk.

Example 14

A five-doctor practice worked from a new build inner city surgery that cost £1.2 million to build. Originally four partners had raised capital of £300k each to buy the building. The fifth partner had decided to stay out of the deal because she was near to retirement anyway. After she retired a new partner joined whose spouse worked for the Foreign Office. He was likely to reach full ambassador status in the next few years, so the new partner could well move on from the practice, and therefore did not wish to buy into the premises.

A few years later one of the partners resigned. He owned part of the building and tried to sell this on to his replacement. However the replacement partner again had good reasons not to buy in. The other partners did not want to have the resigning partner continuing to own a share of the premises, and he did not want to have anything more to do with the practice either. The situation was resolved by the three existing owners extending their capital investment by a further £100k each to buy out the resigning partner. Thus out of five partners, three have a £400k share in the building, whilst two partners feel they have the flexibility they need.

Lease

Leased premises are less of a financial risk as the cost of the lease will normally be covered by payments from the health authority under the rent and rates scheme (covered in Section 51, the most complex of all Red Book sections). Thus, each quarter the landlord is paid the rent on the lease by the practice and the health authority reimburses the practice with a rent payment. Usually, although not invariably, the payments will net out so that the practice neither loses nor gains. However, with lower risk there will be less control over the building and you become subject to the terms of the lease. For example, you might have to completely redecorate every year at the practice's expense.

As the lease is a shared responsibility of the partnership as a whole, and not of individual partners as individual capital investments would be, there is no feeling of individuals being tied down. However, only the landlord ever makes any money out of the arrangement.

Example 15

A four-doctor practice moved into a new building worth £900k. The building was owned by a developer who had financed the project and worked on the design with the partners. Rent was agreed at £90k per year which was paid by the practice to the developer and from the health authority to the practice. Routine maintenance is dealt with by the practice, and paid for out of a rent supplement which the health authority pays to the practice, so the practice retains some control over the building. There remains some uncertainty about what will happen at the rent review in three years when the developer can increase the rent on the advice of an independent surveyor, but the health authority will have to stick to whatever the then district valuer values the rent at. There may be difficult negotiations. However, the practice has got the building it wanted without being tied down to the risk and commitment of a £900k loan.

Rent

Some practices work in community trust buildings, and pay rent which is reimbursed by the health authority in the same way as described above. There is therefore little or no financial risk to the practice, unless the trust goes bankrupt, and no net cost either. There is therefore room for flexibility for partners to join and leave the practice. Links with primary healthcare team members are likely to be good. However the practice will have no control over the building and how it is serviced. They may have to use trust staff, in a shared switchboard for example, and will be subject to trust managers' decisions about the building. There may also be a service charge which is not reimbursed by the health authority.

> *Example 16*
> A three-doctor practice working in a trust health centre wanted to put up some shelving in the practice library. They were faced with a delay of five months whilst the trust decided whether it could agree to this request, as it constituted a change in the building. Bizarre!

Financial issues

In this section we will look at issues related to how practice income is shared out and managed. This is a key part of the partnership deed.

Shares

Rather than draw a fixed salary, a partner takes a share of the practice profits, the money left in the practice after all income and practice expenses including salaries are paid out. This will vary from month to month but a good accountant should be able to predict fairly accurately what your share will turn out to be. Drawings are paid to the partner each month and are worked out to be roughly one-twelfth of the predicted yearly profit.

Some of your profit will be held back each month to build up a tax reserve. Because partners are self-employed they pay tax in two lumps each year, in January and July, based on the previous year's earnings declared in the practice accounts to the tax office in the annual partnership tax return. This sounds complicated, and it is. Never be tempted to sort out your own tax affairs, even when they talk about self-assessment. Pay an accountant to deal with all of this, unless you are an accountant. They will help you with all the forms and advise on what personal expenses (such as car costs and home computer costs) that you can claim against your income to reduce your tax liability. They will also advise about keeping records for seven years and how to log car usage.

Profit shares are usually equal for equal-time partners, but an allowance for part-timers needs to be made. Exactly what share a part-timer draws may be an issue for debate, because it is very hard to measure workload accurately and fairly, especially if partners have different styles and different patients.

Pooling income

A basic decision to be made is what income will be divided up in partnership shares and what will be divided up in different ways. Most of the income will be pooled. That is to say it is put into a central pot where it is set against expenses, to calculate profit which is shared out in profit-sharing ratios. Some income, however, may not be shared out in this way, and this income is called 'prior shares' because it is shared out, in proportions not related to partnership shares, prior to the calculation of profit. For example, if two out of four partners own the building, then the health authority rent income would almost certainly go as a prior share to the owning partners, in proportion to their share of ownership of the building. This would go to offset their mortgage costs. This is fine as the non-owning partners have no financial interest in the building or claim on the rent. However, if the partnership as a whole owned a lease on the building, the rent would go into the pool, and be offset against the cost of the lease which would be paid out of the practice pool. These examples are simple, but some income streams could reasonably be pooled or kept as prior shares depending on your point of view. So earnings from a partner's outside post as a clinical assistant could be kept as a prior share, because that partner does the work, or it could be shared in the pool because during the time the partner is being a clinical assistant, the other partners have to do his practice work on his behalf. There are no firm rules, only what you negotiate.

Which aspects of the practice income will be pooled, and therefore shared out in profit-sharing ratios, and which will be retained individually by partners? Seniority payments are often taken as prior shares, although younger partners may not see why older colleagues should not pool this income. PGEA may be pooled, but would it be fair if a lazy partner who never did any education should bring down everyone's income? Should the minor surgery partner keep all the minor surgery income, or should this be shared out? Some practices pool everything, some divide things in very complex ways to meet individual circumstances.

Attitude to outside work

A particular problem is what to do with income from outside appointments such as clinical assistantships, course organiser appointments, insurance or police work and nursing home retainers. If you pool income, will you redistribute the practice work accordingly so that income reflects workload? It would be unfair to pool a partner's nursing home retainer but insist that she continues to do the same amount of workload within the practice. Another problem arises when time spent on an outside job earns less than could be earned from surgery work. For example, a fee for running an education workshop would be far less than the income generated if the time were spent doing liquid nitrogen minor surgery.

Does the partnership want outside appointments at all? Some practices do not allow it. They can generate a lot of income but also a lot of disruption to surgery work and patient care. Being a police surgeon is said (perhaps by those who do not know) to be a licence to print money, but can mean going out without notice at night or mid-surgery for an indefinite period. There might have to be locum cover for this which may be more expensive than the money you earn. Some appointments, for example course organiser, are relatively poorly paid as well as being time-consuming. Could you put up with a partner doing this?

Outside work may be done in practice time with re-jigging of the workload, or may be done outside practice time. Either way there are issues about who covers the routine surgery work.

Example 17
In a five-doctor practice, outside appointments of the partners include educational and nursing home appointments. Income from these is pooled, but the partners with the appointments do one surgery per week fewer than the others to compensate.

Example 18
In a four-doctor practice the partners each do seven surgeries per week. Outside appointments include occupational health and hospital practitioner posts. These sessions are done in addition to practice work and so the income is not shared.

Pooling expenses

Just as income may or may not be pooled, so also with expenses to a lesser extent. Main practice expenses, for example salaries of staff, will usually come out of the pooled income, but what about more personal things like Medical Defence Union/Medical Protection Society (MDU/MPS) expenses or car expenses when individual partners may be able to get different deals? Partners will probably not all want to drive the same type of car, and different cars cost different amounts so why should partners share out the expenses equally? What about course fees and professional memberships? The fair answer will depend on how you divide up income such as PGEA. You could argue that the practice will pay General Medical Council (GMC) registration fees as it is a flat rate fee per doctor and you have a mutual interest in ensuring that each other's registration is paid.

Usually it is possible to be able to reach reasonable agreement on expenses issues, but it is easy to see how the partnership deed could become quite detailed.

Example 19
A four-doctor practice used a deputising service for night calls. On their nights on call two of the partners did all their own calls

up to midnight and then handed over to the deputising service. Of the other partners, one covered telephone advice only on her evenings on call, and one switched everything over to the deputising service at 7.00 p.m. The partners agreed that the deputising expenses should not be pooled and divided in partnership shares, but should be divided up in proportion to the number of calls done by the service on the nights that each partner was on call. This was an administrative nightmare, not least in keeping track of exactly what use each partner made of the deputising service, but the arrangement did accommodate all the partners' needs.

Sale of good will

If you buy a shop, you would pay for the buildings and stock and other assets, but also, quite properly, for 'good will'. This is the reputation and customer base of the shop, and can be given a monetary value to reflect its importance to the business. In general practice there is an equivalent, and it is illegal. If a single-handed doctor takes on a partner he might say that because everyone knows him and he set up the practice, he should have a larger share of the profits. In effect the new partner is buying 'good will' from the existing partner. This is a form of exploitation. The local medical committees (LMCs) are on the look out for this, even in its hidden form where time or workload is used to buy good will. A senior partner cannot plan to see half as many patients as his partner and claim the same share of the profit. Profit share must always reflect actual workload as far as possible. You can of course be paid more for greater administrative work or greater clinical work. When a new partner joins it is assumed that they will have a lower clinical and, in particular, administrative workload. This is the basis for progression to parity but if progression is too slow, for example more than three years, it will be interpreted as a sale of good will. At all times it should be clear why people are drawing their particular level of share, and it should be obvious to those outside that it is an attempt to reflect work done.

Example 8 revisited
This five-doctor practice used to work with an executive partner system and their partnership shares were weighted so that the executive partner drew a slightly larger share than the others. As the work of the partners changed they swapped to a shared responsibility system. Before long the four previously junior partners realised that the existing partnership shares were not only unjust but could represent an illegal sale of good will. At a tense and frank partnership meeting they confronted the issue and with a unanimous decision they altered the shares to reflect true workload. Having a working knowledge of the legal position certainly helped focus the discussion.

Example 20
Doctor M was hoping to join a four-handed practice and asked at the second interview to see the accounts. He was presented with a brown envelope containing a variety of documentation, including income and expenditure accounts for the previous three months and a handful of bank statements! Despite this evident chaos he joined the practice, and discovered that the culture of colluding to avoid conflict was widespread. No one had wanted to tackle the financial situation because they did not want to admit that they were in over their heads and did not know where to start. Anyway, they all drew a reasonable income each month so there was no perceived pressing need. After partnership changes, practice manager changes and a GP contract change, the practice gradually sorted out its finances through a steady process of education and change management.

Example 21
Doctor N had just finished his registrar year and had been approached to join a local six-partner teaching practice. When he examined the accounts he found high profits as a result of high deprivation payments and item-of-service fees. The accountants

were specialist medical accountants who had produced a commentary on the accounts suggesting ways in which efficiency could be improved. The accounts also showed that a full range of services was being offered. Doctor N was sure that at this practice his financial future would be secure, but he also could see from the high list size that he was going to have to work hard.

Banking policy and accounts

The partnership deed will specify the partnership's bankers (who should be local, for convenience), and accountants (who may or may not be local). There is a lot to be said for using accountants with a special interest in GP accounts, given the complexity of the Red Book. Accountants will sort out yearly accounts (or quarterly if required, at a price) and deal with partnership taxation and offer advice on financial issues if required. Professional fees of accountants vary considerably so it is worth considering inviting quotes from different firms if the bill seems high.

It used to be the case that partners could be held personally liable for any unpaid tax from any partner's share of the profits, but now, under self-assessment, you will only be liable for the tax on your share of the profits. However, each partner can still be held liable for the whole of any other partnership debt if the partnership defaults.

References

1 Neighbour R (1992) *The Inner Apprentice*. Kluwer, Lancaster.
2 Belbin M (1981) *Management Teams: why they succeed or fail*. Butterworth Heinemann, Oxford.
3 Ting-Tooney S and Oetzel JG (2001) *Managing Intercultural Conflict Effectively*. Sage, London.

3

Salaried general practitioners

Peter Aquino and Bhupinder Kohli

The general practitioner (GP) registrar year is a busy period. Registrars are usually so preoccupied with trying to cope with the transition from hospital medicine to general practice and passing summative assessment (SA) that deciding on their next step can often be the last thing on their mind.

Until recently, entering a partnership would have seemed the next logical step, but the new breed of GPs are less willing to make this commitment straight away. The reasons for this are varied and complex but include an unwillingness to have increased responsibility, a desire to travel in the future and the unappealing prospect of committing yourself to one practice for the next 30 years.

Many newly qualified GPs will not have worked at the same job for more than six months, and some will never have worked in the same geographical area for a similar period, so the idea of long-term commitment can be frightening. Many alternatives exist to becoming a GP partner, including working as an associate, a locum, or a salaried GP. Salaried GPs are a new concept and offer a viable and attractive alternative to partnership. With the removal of the old general medical services (GMS) 'partner specific' allowances, the employment of salaried GPs by practices without penalty is a huge incentive for practices.

Unlike the old assistantship, where a GP would be employed by a practice to do a few sessions of specific work, often with low pay and no control over their work, modern salaried work is reasonably paid, and exploitation is squeezed out by standardised terms and conditions and a relative shortage of good candidates being enticed to lots of good jobs. GPs can be employed directly by practices, often using personal medical services (PMS) growth money, or by primary care trusts (PCTs) to work in existing practices, or by PCTs to run specific projects or to set up new practices.

Main differences between salaried GPs and partnership

Advantages

As with every job there are aspects to the work that are appealing and some which are not (Box 3.1). Salaried posts should be attractive to newly qualified GPs who are interested in earning a guaranteed income and practising general practice without getting involved in the business side of the practice. As there is a lot of flexibility in the job this may be particularly suitable if you have to juggle family life and work or if you have interests outside work. Not having a long-term commitment to a practice will allow you to travel to Australia for that long trip you always wanted (once you have saved enough) or just to take a break away from medicine for a while.

Having less paperwork will mean that your practice time is essentially patient-focused. There is also protected study leave and a postgraduate education allowance (PGEA), so your professional development should still continue. Being salaried should also be attractive if you are considering partnership but are just not ready to make a long-term commitment. This option will offer an introduction to a practice before any potential partnership starts. Salaried GPs are not just an 'extra pair of hands', and you should have a clearly defined and important role in your practice.

Box 3.1: Benefits for the salaried GP

Advantages
- Introduction to life as a general practitioner without the business worries.
- Flexibility — no long-term commitment, and working hours can be easily negotiated to suit family or outside work interests.
- Less paperwork and administration than partners.
- Guaranteed income (£5000–£8000 per session per year) depending on scheme.
- Superannuation scheme is maintained.
- Under PMS, salaried GPs employed by a PCT can develop a personal list.
- No equity to bring or financial risk involved.

Disadvantages
- Usually lower income than peers who go into partnership.
- May be viewed by some as 'lower' status than partnership.
- Short-term contract.
- Full maternity and sick pay may have to be negotiated (guaranteed if the salaried GP is employed by a PCT).

A salaried GP may have a personal list but usually only if employed by a PCT (*see* options in a salaried scheme below), rather than by a practice where the personal list will usually be under one of the partners. It still may be possible to have a personal list if employed by a practice, but this would have to be negotiated. Some GPs may like the idea of having a personal list, although it may bring added responsibility.

Disadvantages

Salaried posts do have some disadvantages. The salary will probably be higher as a partner, and this could be important if you are looking to enter into the property market or finally pay off your student debts. Being salaried may be perceived by some as a 'lower' status than partnership (in much the same way that the pinnacle of hospital medicine may be perceived by some as the consultant rather than a staff grade post).

Support on a salaried scheme can be variable, and it is wise to choose a post where good support will be offered. The support that a salaried general practitioner should expect is in the form of a post-vocational training scheme (VTS) style afternoon where salaried GPs can get together and discuss educational and other issues. Importantly, it also provides a social network. In some salaried schemes this afternoon will be paid for. A partnership may offer better long-term security as it is much harder to dispense with a partner than a salaried GP, and the contract for the salaried GP is usually short-term, for example two to three years. After this time a salaried GP may wish to go into partnership or decide to choose another area to work in. With the current crisis in GP recruitment, if a salaried GP wished to renew their contract it would probably be fairly easy to do.

In short, if you are considering a partnership but are not quite sure, it may be wise to be a salaried GP for a year or so before making your final decision. It may well be that in the future all potential partnerships will have an option of a one-year salaried post.

Options in a salaried scheme

The options in the salaried scheme include working as a salaried GP to a practice or to a PCT. There are very important differences between these two posts. If you are a salaried GP employed by a PCT you may work in one or two practices within the trust's area, whereas if you are employed by a particular practice you will only work for that practice. Importantly, if you are salaried and work for a PCT you will be entitled to defined holiday and study leave, receive full maternity and sick pay, and be paid according to a Whitley council pay scale. If you are employed by a practice, however, the above have to be negotiated, but a good practice will have no problems if you want to peg terms and conditions to the local PCT contract at least. You may also have to negotiate hours of work and reimbursement of medical indemnity and protection fees, and BMA subscription and course fees. Also, as a practice is a much smaller organisation to deal with than a PCT, any queries regarding pay or other issues can be dealt with much more quickly.

Other salaried options include posts which include academic sessions such as the London academic training scheme (LATS) and post-VTS jobs (also known as senior registrar jobs). The former is ideal if you are interested in research or academia as the work is split between clinical commitments, developing research skills and under-taking a project. The post-VTS jobs are great if you have a special interest in a particular area as these jobs allow you to develop skills in that field. For example, in our trust one senior registrar is devel-oping skills in cognitive behaviour therapy as well as having normal clinical work. These posts can be negotiated through your local deanery and usually consist of half the GP's time being spent in normal clinical work and the other half in his or her specialised field. However a general practice senior registrar (GPSR) job will be limited to six months only, and is paid at the rate of a registrar with suitable increment. Also, if you take a GPSR post you will not get your Joint Committee on Postgraduate Training for General Practice (JCPTGP) certificate until the end of the job, so your 'Golden Hello' will be delayed and any later time-served related benefits (such as senior-ity and approval as a trainer) may also be delayed. You also cannot do locum work as a GPSR.

You might find that a PCT salaried job will allow you sessions to learn specific skills, especially if you can convince them that it will help you develop skills as a GP with a special interest. Occasionally practice-based jobs may offer this. One of our local practices with strong educational skills offers a post with five clinical sessions and two sessions for specific and supervised educational work, such as working for Membership of the Royal College of General Practi-tioners (MRCGP) or working for publications designed for a new GP wanting to bridge the gap between GP registrar (GPR) and fully self-reliant practitioner.

Points to consider when applying for jobs

Many advertisements in the medical press are well written and have attractive pictures attached to them but do they tell the full story? Below are listed several pointers to questions to ask when consid-ering a new practice.

- Is the salary what you are looking for?
- Are the working conditions suitable for you?
- Is a mentor and induction period provided?
- Is self-directed learning encouraged?
- What efforts do the practice make so that you feel part of the 'team'?
- Are they flexible for any specific requests, e.g childcare, holidays?
- Will the practice give full maternity and sick pay?
- Is there the possibility of becoming a partner after a period of being salaried?

Personal experience

Peter Aquino

I have worked as a salaried GP in East London for the past two years. I really enjoyed my registrar year so I stayed on at the same practice for a further year. There were five registrars on my VTS. Two went into partnership straight away, two of us became salaried, and the other has left general practice altogether.

As I am pursuing a career in primary care epidemiology, being a salaried GP was a way of gaining experience as a 'fully fledged' GP for a year without getting involved in the business aspect of the practice. I liked the idea of flexibility, and I was very fortunate in that my practice allowed me to choose my working hours to suit my academic interests. Effectively, I undertook the same amount of clinical work as the partners (same number of patients per surgery and number of house visits) but did not get involved in any business decisions. This meant that I had less paperwork. I still had a say in the clinical aspects of the practice and felt an integral part of the practice and in no way a 'lesser' GP than any of the partners.

My second salaried post has been even more flexible. In university term times I do academic study, but still need an income. I work full-time in the holidays. My practice-based salaried contract averages out the clinical work I do over the course of the year and pays me regularly each month as if I were part-time all year. So I get a regular income and fit in the work when I can.

Summary

Salaried GPs may help reduce the workload and burden on busy pressurised practices. New blood can bring fresh ideas that ultimately should benefit both practices and patients by producing a new group of confident, clinically astute GPs who are willing to continue in life-long learning and development. This may have a 'knock on' effect and encourage older principals to further their education and development too. With the current difficulties in general practice recruitment and retention, salaried posts may be one way in which this current trend is reversed.

4

Locums

Lise Hertel

The life of a locum! Young, free and single! No ties, vast amounts of money, pick and choose work as you wish, stay in bed when you want to! Is it really as good as all that? It can be for the right person. Why do people choose to become locums? Those just out of their registrar year often want to look around different practices before deciding where to settle, or maybe they may choose to be a locum because it means that you can drop everything at a moment's notice and travel the world or grasp that job which you have been waiting for. More experienced general practitioners (GPs) may choose it because they have had enough of being tied to a partnership, because their partner is in a job that requires moving around a lot or because they have retired but just want to do a little work to remember the old days without the strain! However, others choose it as a long-term career option.

The advantages

As with every job there is good stuff and bad stuff. Being a locum is wonderful because you can work when you want to and where you want to. I know of doctors who work full-time two weeks on and then have two weeks off, which enables them to work anywhere in the country for the best pay, but allows their families to live where they wish — where it is cheaper, in the country or maybe where the best schools are. I have worked with people who fly into remote islands around the British Isles to do a week or two as a locum, sample the local cuisine and do some fishing or sailing. (Remote practices will often pay your travel expenses making this a fun and inexpensive option.) You can have a part-time permanent locum for a year (say mornings only) and dabble in afternoon locums when the fancy takes you, or you need the money! Often you may even get a choice of surgery times, particularly if you negotiate before you start, for example a 9.30 a.m. start so you can get the kids to school or 3–5 p.m. to be able to get to that yoga class, favour-ite pub or religious event! You must be firm but fair when setting up a locum with a practice, insisting on a contract before you start, or, as many locums do, bringing your own contract with you and agreeing it with the practice manager before you start. (This of course can also be done by email or fax the day or week before if there is time.)

Most good practices will send you a locum pack before you arrive (although any longer than 10 pages gets to be rather a lot of read-ing!). Some are useful, some have not been updated since the year dot and, worst of all, some are given to you as you arrive! You then have to fumble through it every time you need some information!

Most doctors I know who work as locums agree that two of the best aspects of the job are that you see a lot of real medicine — regu-lar patients usually save themselves for their regular doctors — and you get to see more new presentations and emergencies. In addition to this, when you turn up for a locum people are nearly always glad to see you!

Box 4.1: Advantages of being a locum

- Flexibility.
- Money (the going rate in London at the moment is £85 an hour and rising!).
- No managerial and staff responsibilities.

- Often have the opportunity to do more 'real' medicine as the 'heart-sinks' either go to their regular GPs or wait until they are back from holiday.
- Can turn work down.
- Can charge for what you do.
- Everyone is grateful when you turn up, making you feel really wanted and appreciated!
- Work where you want, when you want.
- Opportunity to see how different practices work, and to look around for a partnership if that is what you are after.
- Can often choose the times of your surgeries.

The disadvantages

Along with the good stuff there has to be bad stuff as well! Depending where you are in your life you may not have any debts or financial worries but if you have a mortgage, car loan or a student debt to pay off then you need to know where your next pay cheque is coming from. Therefore as a locum you constantly need to be thinking ahead. Where will I be next week, next month, next year? Sometimes different locums do not fit together very well and this can require a lot of phone calls and negotiation so that all parties are happy. For example, can I start my surgery at 8.30 a.m. so I will finish and have time to drive for an hour to get to my afternoon locum? You want a maternity locum from February to September? Oh dear, I cannot do that but I could offer April to September – would this be any good? And so on and so on. Some people enjoy the challenge of this and some people find it a bind!

There is also the problem of seasonal variation in demand. Everyone wants you for the holidays and not so much in the autumn. This can interfere with your own holiday plans, especially if you have school-age children. The choice is lose money or miss your holiday. Of course there is no holiday pay as a locum and this has to be planned for.

Contracts can be difficult. We do not get much training in employment law as doctors, but if you plan to be a locum for some time it is well worth thinking about what a session means to you. Is it two hours face-to-face surgery and two hours clear-up time? Or is it two and a half hours face-to-face and clear-up, or maybe 20 patients, three phone calls and a visit? This is very important to get clear because some surgeries have no boundaries and work four-hour face-to-face surgeries before they get to the visits and the phone calls! Others are very strict about numbers in a booked surgery, but watch out for the emergency surgery that can add 10 patients to your list! Advanced access has also added to the headache. The practice may have worked out its day-to-day demand, but as we all know people are like buses — sometimes they all come at once! How much will you help out? How much more money will you ask for, and have you included this in your locum contract?

Getting paid is very important — *very important*. Life is busy enough without endlessly having to chase money you are owed from months ago. Contracts give you some protection, but who wants to enforce one through a solicitor or small claims court? For most short-term locums it is better for everyone if the cheque is waiting for you at the end of the session, or at the end of the week — job done!

After getting paid, paying your tax and National Insurance (NI) are the most important points. To be a successful locum you must be well organised and logical and you need an accountant who understands about general practice and what you can and cannot claim for. Alternatively there are some great software packages for the self-employed (Microsoft Money, for example) and doing your tax return online can be very helpful. Those lovely people at the tax office stay open until 10 p.m. at night, which is very useful for those last minute questions before the deadline. Many locums choose to keep a separate high-earnings saving account to save for their tax bill. This is a good idea and a great stress reliever!

Getting paid and organising tax and NI are not the only reasons why being a successful locum means being well organised. If you have children, or even a dog that needs walking, dropping everything and rushing off to do a last minute locum an hour away is just not an option. Who will pick your children up? Will the dog have eaten your kitchen table by the time you get home? Some people have wonderful parents and friends who will step in at a moment's notice — some do not.

Constant switching between IT systems, and more importantly how much different practices use their IT systems, for example paperless, paperlight, stone-age man, etc., can be a bit tiring! And don't even think about passwords! Good practices will organise it before you come, but others may just forget until you have arrived and no one can remember and the senior partner is out of contact! However, these problems can be managed by taking more long-term locums and fewer short or single sessions. Also there is all the boring but very necessary stuff such as referral forms (where are they?), who to refer to and the inevitable mysterious mental health teams — who are they, where are they? It is always different wherever you go!

Then there is always the missing dictaphone! This is the same almost anywhere you go, and if there is one there is usually no tape! Of course no locum would not mention the downside of working in a male doctor's room (even if you are male); there is hardly ever any female equipment, which means you have to go out to reception and ask for the whereabouts of a speculum and explain what it is for, and then there is some giggling and a suggestion that maybe you might find it in the nurse's room. And it is unusual if you do not get given the smallest room, hot in summer and cold in winter, and a printer that was old before the ark set sail and either jams all the time or does not work at all! A friend told me he had to work in a room so small that to examine the patient he had to stand up, push in his chair and allow the patient to squeeze past to the examination couch, and then any patient over five feet did not fit on anyway and had to bend their legs! Sometimes it is just a challenge finding room to work amongst the absent partner's paperwork! It is always important to discover the whereabouts of the toilet before starting surgery — both for you and the patients!

A chapter on being a locum would not be complete without a mention of parking. If you choose only to work in practices with car parks then you will have no problems (until you go on a home visit that is!), but most of us have received numerous tickets. (The more generous surgeries pay them for you and seem to recognise it is a risk a locum takes.) I know of someone who only just managed to talk his way out of a clamp when he was parked outside a patient's house doing a visit! It does not make for a relaxing surgery when you have to rush to the window between patients to check that your car is still there and not sporting an attractive yellow shoe!

Not to be forgotten is the fact that you have no job security. Apart from no holiday pay, there is no study leave and, this is very important, no sick pay. If you are going to locum get good sick pay cover, and maybe medical insurance if you can afford it. Even a broken wrist in a skiing accident or an ingrowing toenail can set you back a few thousand pounds!

Finally there is temptation and greed! Yes, it *is* true, there is always work for a locum. You could work 365 days a year, 24 hours a day if you choose. You could earn £200–250k easily but will you have a life? Will you crack under the strain? Or will you end up a millionaire, owning several houses and cars, and paying off your friends' mortgages? There is also the temptation to work because people are begging you; they are desperate; they have not been on holiday since they started as a GP; they ring you up and beg you to work, just this once. Often they are people that you know and you want to help them. However, remember you are not the only locum in the world, and you must look after yourself too. Your income depends on it!

Box 4.2: The disadvantages of being a locum

- Insecurity – where will your next job be?
- Lack of contracts – often the goal posts are moved at the last moment.
- Tax – don't underestimate this! Be well organised.
- Sending invoices and chasing cheques – best to insist on payment at the end of each session or a week before leaving the building!
- Planning – if you have children it can be difficult to drop everything and get to that early morning last minute job.
- Variation and demand – everyone wants you in the summer!
- Constant switching between IT systems, methods of referral/ request forms, etc.
- Mental Health Services – they are different in each area and usually referral pathways are mysterious!
- Parking tickets – don't get me started on those!
- Dictaphones – where are they all?
- Male doctor rooms – there is never any female equipment!
- Printers – usually the worst and the oldest!
- Temptation to work more than is good for you.
- No sick or holiday pay.

Summary

It might seem after the last section of this chapter that being a locum is not all it is cracked up to be, and perhaps the huge rise in the pay of salaried GPs will soon make it a less favourable option, but at present it is still a great way to earn money and see general practice, warts and all, with no commitment and just a little bit of adventure. Who knows what the next locum will be? Who you will meet? And what opportunities will come your way?

5

Academic general practice

Sally Hull and Peter Aquino

For any newly qualified general practitioner (GP) who is interested in the idea of developing the skills for research and teaching, an academic career may seem the way forward.

These days there are a number of routes into an academic career. Although the term is usually associated with university departments, research is by no means confined to universities. The expansion of medical schools has meant that much more teaching is based in practices during both the community or general practice modules, and also more broadly throughout the medical curriculum.

So the first question to ask yourself is what are you most interested in doing. Do you want to become an undergraduate teacher, or do you want to become a researcher? Also you will need to consider whether you want to pursue the academic component as your primary career path, or whether you want to be a clinician with a special interest in research or teaching.

University-based academic general practice

The first University Department of General Practice was founded in Edinburgh in 1957, with the first professor being appointed in 1963. Other universities were slow to follow this lead, with the first chair in England being founded in Manchester in 1972. Every undergraduate medical school in the UK now has an academic Department of General Practice or Department of Primary Care, although many of them have functioned with an unsatisfactory level of infrastructure and a low number of tenured posts. Recently, there has been a move to blur the boundaries between departments, and for research teams to work across interdisciplinary boundaries in a confederation of community health science disciplines. Other key developments have been extending the boundaries of departments into the community by working in partnership with networks of research and teaching practices.

General practice and primary care remain at the heart of decision making in the NHS, with 90% of patient encounters taking place there. The opportunities for research are endless, and over the last 30 years there has been a great expansion of research both based in practice – exploring the content and delivery of care – and based on primary care – exploring the organisation of services. The opportunities still remain, as general practice changes in response to new developments and changing social patterns; the only thing which is certain will be our need to explore new areas of uncertainty.

In 1997 the report of an independent task force on *Clinical Academic Careers* in the UK[1] found that almost every department had difficulty recruiting staff in general practice. This was largely due to historic low levels of research capacity, a lack of systematic training and career pathways for academic staff, and an adverse funding arrangement which meant that full-time clinical practice was likely to be better financially rewarded than an academic career. At a national level the response has been to develop the National Primary Care Awards scheme. This is run by the NHS research and development programme to identify the most able individuals who wish to pursue a career in primary care research, providing financial and training support. Locally, many departments have expanded access to research training, and postgraduate studentships for those wishing to pursue an MD or PhD. A research doctorate is an essential grounding for those who want to become the future senior academics in universities.

Practice-based teaching opportunities (Box 5.1)

Box 5.1: Jubilee Street Practice, Tower Hamlets, population 9300

A hub teaching practice for Barts and The London, Queen Mary's School of Medicine and Dentistry. The practice has a contract to provide 85 undergraduate teaching sessions annually. These include sessions during the medical, paediatric, obstetric and gynaecology modules as well as the community modules and special study modules.

Benefits
- New challenge and job variety.
- Refreshment of teachers' knowledge base.
- Training and support for teaching.
- Financial support – may include infrastructure funding and sessional payments.
- Opportunities to build further links with academic departments to develop teaching, and to become involved in educational research and other projects.

Disadvantages
- Teaching may conflict with clinical responsibilities at busy times.
- Teaching income is lower than from clinical practice.

Developing academic skills from general practice

Many doctors at the beginning of their career are not sure which career path they want to take. The climate in general practice has never been so good for those who want to have a taste of different options. This is in marked contrast to the situation 20 years ago when most GPs had a rather static career pathway unless they actively sought out the unusual. These days a CV which includes a variety of posts will demonstrate that you have equipped yourself with a range of skills to broaden your portfolio.

Salaried GP schemes with academic sessions

The young GP who has finished vocational training and is interested in exploring an academic option should definitely consider some of the salaried posts offered by primary care trusts (PCTs). Many of these have been developed with an eye to local recruitment and retention and may include academic sessions. These may be linked to a department of general practice and offer the GP opportunities to join a project team, or develop teaching skills. Some will offer the chance to do a modular MSc in primary care, which will include structured teaching on research methods and a project report or dissertation. Some posts include sessions attached to a hospital department. These may provide research opportunities in a well resourced and research active department. On the other hand they may be a cover for basic service provision.

Another scheme which provides an excellent starter is the post-vocational, or senior registrar post. This is usually a six-month post combining clinical sessions and an attachment of your choice. It is tailor-made, and demands some planning to gain a suitable attachment or supervisor. These schemes can be moulded to provide an introduction to academic practice. Whether or not you pursue an academic career you will have gained a new range of skills, and the confidence to make your next career move.

Becoming a GP with a special interest in research

Many GPs at the start of their career want to spend the first few years based entirely in clinical practice and gaining experience in practice management. At some point in the career of most GPs there will come a time when they feel a need to broaden their career.

Indeed research has shown that stress and burn-out tend to be less in those doctors who do not work full-time as clinicians with front-line responsibility for patients. Research is one of a growing number of special interests which can be developed. Reasons for starting vary widely. Many doctors become fascinated by a particular clinical or organisational problem which they want to research. Others want to gain skills in appraising literature for changing their clinical practice, or become involved through teaching registrars or undergraduates.

There are many routes into an academic training. Perhaps the most popular at present is to do an MSc, either as a day-release from clinical practice, or as a full-time taught course during a period of sabbatical leave from the practice. Sabbatical leave, funded by the prolonged study leave arrangement, will still be available when the new general medical services (GMS) contract starts in 2004. For novice researchers it is essential to get basic training in the variety of research methods – undertaking a literature search, quantitative and qualitative data analysis, and in the mechanics of writing a project grant, gaining ethics approval and satisfying research governance procedures.

An alternative route is to make links with a local primary care research network. These can usually provide a mentor to help develop a project, often some bursary funding to start the process, and a local community of researchers with whom to share your progress.

Box 5.2 lists some of the ways GPs may get started in research.

Box 5.2: Ways to get started in research

The post-VTS GP
- Join a salaried post with academic sessions.
- Consider a salaried post with the opportunity to do an MSc in primary care.
- Apply for a senior registrar post with an academic supervisor.
- Do a full-time MSc in a subject of your choice.
- Apply for a post as lecturer in a university department.

The GP in practice
- Do an MSc based in a university department, by reducing your clinical commitments.

- Take a sabbatical to do a full-time course or project.
- Join a local research network.
- Take advice on your career move from a senior academic.

Research practices and primary care research networks

During the 1990s the Department of Health saw a need to increase the research capacity in primary care organisations (PCOs).

The first research practice was appointed in 1994 by the Royal College of General Practitioners (RCGP) and given some limited infrastructure funding to provide the administrative support required for a practice to set up as a serious research unit. Following this example some research networks have given funding to support research active practices, and the RCGP has underpinned this with an accreditation scheme aimed at good practice in research management and governance. Many networks will also give bursaries to support practitioners who need protected time to develop a project. Other large networks include the Medical Research Council's General Practice Research Framework with a membership of 1000 practices which collect data for large epidemiological studies.

Networks have contributed a great deal to promoting evidence-based practice and research as an activity for primary care practitioners. They have contributed to research methods training, and have done a number of studies which have emerged from the questions of practising clinicians.

From 2004, PCTs will have a central role in managing research governance within their locality. The role they will play in commissioning, funding and supporting primary care research in the future remains unclear.

Personal experience

Peter Aquino

My road into academic general practice was purely accidental. I had left medical school intent on becoming an inner city GP. However, after having completed my house jobs and accident and emergency post I decided I needed a career break. I undertook some research involving developing a method for analysing brain volumes using magnetic resonance imaging (MRI) techniques. I found this research very stimulating, but still felt that I lacked the necessary research foundation skills. I received a Medical Research Council (MRC) studentship to pursue an MPhil in epidemiology which essentially taught me the necessary skills to undertake academic research. I then went back and finished my GP training and since then have undergone further advanced training in medical statistics. My route into this area has been rather unconventional, but I have the best of three worlds – clinical contact with patients, teaching and research. This means I do not get bored, I have a life and one that is very rewarding.

Summary

The opportunities for developing an academic component to a career in general practice have never been so good. There is a wide range of pathways into academic training, many of which are seen as important elements in the recruitment and retention of a scarce workforce. In the future every GP should be able to develop a special interest as part of their professional development, and for some it will be research.

Reference

1 Committee of Vice Chancellors and Principals (1997) *Clinical Academic Careers. Report of an independent task force.* CVCP, London.

6

Postgraduate education

Petre Jones

For historical reasons postgraduate medical education is dealt with by deaneries and is quite separate from research departments and undergraduate education. This emphasises the fact that the skills of research are different from the skills of teaching. Some people are skilled at both but many prefer one approach over the other. For me teaching is fascinating, but research seems slow and distant, and so I have concentrated on developing a career in medical education rather than academia.

The role of the trainer is to spend an intensive year on a one-to-one basis working with a colleague as they pass through one of the major transitions of the medical world, from junior hospital, illness-focused doctor to independent community and patient-focused doctor. Each general practice registrar (GPR) who takes that journey does it differently and needs different support, and has a different impact on the trainer and the practice. Other educational roles are also interesting and challenging but most people start in the world of postgraduate education by becoming a trainer. So, this chapter looks in some detail at how to become a trainer, and in less detail at the other major postgraduate educational roles that you may come across and aspire to.

The structure of postgraduate education (Figure 6.1)

Each deanery has a slightly different central deanery structure but will have, in principle, a dean of postgraduate education for general practice, working full-time in the post. They are responsible for the strategic management of the deanery and coordinating with other deans at national level. Around them is a team of deputy deans, associate deans, and task orientated associate deans (TOADS). They do the actual job of running the deanery and the educational structures within the deanery. Each will have lead responsibility for issues relating to a particular geographical patch, or lead on a particular project or set of issues, such as summative assessment (SA). Supported by them are the people who actually deliver the education – trainers, course organisers (COs), higher professional education (HPE) directors and deanery tutors, working in every district, facilitating different aspects of postgraduate education.

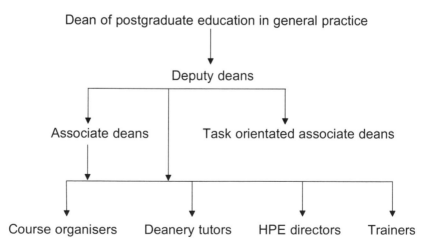

Figure 6.1   The structure of postgraduate education

The trainer

The trainer's role

The trainer's role may seem fairly obvious, to provide practice based education in tutorials and clinical support for the GPR. They also need to be able to manage educational-related issues in the practice to make sure standards are kept up, and they must carry enough weight within the practice to ensure, for example, that the GPR is not asked to do inappropriate work.

However, there are other roles apart from purely being a teacher. The trainer may act as mentor, helping the GPR reflect on the changes they are passing through, and sometime act as a shoulder to cry on. They may have to feed back challenging stuff which is difficult to hear, and on the odd bizarre occasion do weird stuff. One trainer I know, with a first tutorial with a new GPR, who casually mentioned he was house-hunting, said 'Let's go and buy you a flat' – so they did, there and then. A good trainer will define their role in terms of the needs of the GPR, rather than follow a preset curriculum, or worse still think only in terms of SA or Membership of the Royal College of General Practitioners (MRCGP).

So why be a trainer?

Box 6.1: Advantages of becoming a trainer

- Education is fun!
- Training is a good way to keep one's own knowledge and clinical skills base up to date, and challenge old assumptions.
- GPRs are placed in practices for their own educational needs and are supernumerary to the practice, which should be able to manage okay without them, but having someone conducting about 3000 consultations per year, and thereby learning, makes a big hole in the mountain of practice workload, and the deanery even pays their salary. Mind you, the workload of teaching will largely fill up this hole again!
- Training is a challenge. It is by no means easy to be a good trainer, and most of us thrive on a challenging and worthwhile

task. As such, becoming a trainer can refresh a doctor with a new interest, perhaps after five or ten years of working in the same role.

- Regular deanery inspections ensure that the training practice has to keep to the standards set by the deanery, This was recognised when sustained quality allowance, under the old general medical services (GMS) contract, was automatically awarded to training practices.
- Trainers get to attend regular trainers' workshops to share problems and learn new skills.

Box 6.2: Disadvantages of becoming a trainer

- *Cost*   It is expensive to become a trainer, especially if premises need to be altered to create a new consulting room for example. Even without this, there will be video equipment to buy, the costs of a new library, locum costs as you go on new teachers' courses and some new clinical equipment to get. When I became a trainer in 1996, we estimated it had cost £14k. With the trainer's grant (the amount the trainer actually gets paid for the year of training a GPR) at £6.6k, it is clear that you will not get rich quick as a trainer.
- *Space*   Training takes space, for a library and for the GPR to consult and study; if this space is not available you will have to build.
- *Organisation*   Your practice manager will have to learn new skills and master the web of administration if the practice is to get reimbursement for the GPR salary.
- *Time*   The trainer needs to spend the equivalent of two sessions training, one for a tutorial and the other spread over the week as hot topic teaching and support.
- Having an inexperienced doctor in the practice carries some clinical risk which has to be managed, although after 11 GPRs I have never had a significant clinical problem arising out of the actions of a GPR. It is really about the trainer offering enough support and availability to talk about difficult patients and problems. Having said that, a GPR who is difficult can become a real nightmare for the trainer.

- *Courses* Becoming a trainer involves going on training course and update days. This takes time and locum costs, although most such courses are in the end very worthwhile.

Pathway to becoming a trainer

The deanery will have a long list of practice and doctor requirements, so contacting the deanery is a good place to start. This is a list of the key highlights, and the ones that usually create difficulties.

The doctor

- You will need to have been in the practice for three years if it is already a training practice or five years for a new training practice, but you can start the application process before this. You might wish to start your educationalist career by teaching medical students, initially on a one-to-one basis, or doing sessions with continuing professional development meetings or on the vocational training scheme (VTS).
- The prospective trainer will have to pass MRCGP. This is a national requirement and could be done by assessment of practice or by examination.
- You will then have to attend a deanery basic trainers' course (or new teachers' course). In London this now runs over 12 days, which is a lot of locums.
- You will then have to work out in your practice how training will work, and what tools you will use.
- Start going to the trainers' workshop.

The practice

Becoming a training practice should be considered a whole team process, and all the team should be actively involved in training the GPR.

- The practice should look in detail at the deanery requirements and plan an implementation strategy and time line.

- Getting all the notes summarised is often a problem, but the primary care trust (PCT) may give you some money to employ a notes summariser. Overseas doctors studying for the Professional and Linguistic Assessments' Board (PLAB) test are often happy to do this work, and nurses are easily trained. However, it is quite possible for non-medical people to be trained to summarise. I have used a geography undergraduate and a Cambridge classics graduate who used to teach as summarisers, and even a 15-year-old school student to summarise immunisation and cervical smear data under close supervision.
- Premises   The GPR will ideally need their own room and there needs to be space for a library and tutorials. You might have to convert rooms, or you may have to build.
- Another thing to develop is a library. There is nothing for it but to get the deanery book list and buy some books. You could go round the bookshops, or go to the *BMJ* bookshop on the net. A budget of about £1000 will get you a reasonable start-off library, and this cost will be recouped after two months of the first GPR's trainers grant. (Oh the joy of spending £1000 in one go on books!)

The inspection

Finally after all this you will be ready to ask the deanery to visit. It might be worth asking the course organisers to do a dummy visit first.

Your local associate dean will visit the practice with a team, which may include another trainer, a practice nurse and a practice manager. They will spend a whole afternoon interviewing various members of the practice team and looking at how the practice works. They will then recommend, or not, to the deanery to appoint you as a trainer. *Hot tip*: it is a good idea to have some nice cakes or nibbles to offer the visitors. A bit of pre-visit detective work should determine the associate dean's favourite.

Thinking of becoming a trainer?

Never take the decision to become a trainer lightly. As you have read, it will impact not only on you but your practice and possibly even your family, with time commitments taken into consideration. Before making any decision reflect on some of the attributes needed which are listed below. If these apply to you then discuss with your practice and family that you are thinking of becoming a trainer and *go for it!*

Attributes of a good trainer

- Approachability.
- Honesty.
- Enthusiasm about teaching.
- Patience.
- Patient-centredness in consultations.

Personal experience

I wanted to become a trainer right from my days as a registrar. My own trainer was inspirational, not least in her patience, and I viewed being a trainer as the highest grade of GP. I joined a non-training practice and passed the MRCGP. After three years as a partner I went on the deanery basic trainers' course, although had to wait a whole year to get a place. Then came the process of getting the practice up to scratch. We converted a small group room into a consulting room next to mine and topped up the practice library. Summarising was a problem; the branch surgery had already got all the notes summarised, but the main surgery was a problem. I trained a geography student to summarise notes and she managed 500 very satisfactorily before falling ill. I then bit the bullet and summarised the remaining 5000 myself over 13 weeks. After a delay due to a change in associate dean, eventually we were visited and, as was standard then, interviewed on a separate occasion. It took two and a half years from applying to become a trainer to finally being approved. Sadly, within a month of approval the deanery were looking to close our VTS because of small numbers and a retiring CO. Determined to keep the scheme going for the sake of the existing trainees, and to ensure my work so far was not wasted, I volunteered to apply to be a job share CO. My first GPR started after I was appointed as a CO, and so began for me the two educational jobs that still grip me.

Course organising

Unlike trainers, who are self-employed as part of their practice work, COs are directly employed on the deanery pay roll at a nationally negotiated pay rate. Most work in small groups running VTS schemes, although arrangements vary between deaneries. They are appointed after an application process and usually fill existing vacancies. Occasionally, completely new posts are funded. COs are usually appointed from the existing local trainers.

Box 6.3: Advantages of course organising

- You not only get to organise the scheme but you have un-limited opportunities to teach within the group setting.
- It is hard work and enormous fun, especially on residentials.
- You get to work with a whole group of colleagues in the educational process.
- You develop small group skills and management skills that will be useful in the practice.
- Raising the profile of the practice with GPRs will help when trying to recruit new doctors and locum cover to the practice.
- It offers the chance to develop something worthwhile.

Box 6.4: Disadvantages of course organising

- As ever in education there is not enough time or money involved to do what you would really like.
- Opportunities to become a CO are limited.

Higher professional education (HPE) directors and deanery tutors

These people are again employed directly by the deanery. They usually already have a background in GP postgraduate education.

HPE directors deal with doctors in the first two years after finishing training, in the period known as higher professional training, facilitating learning around the special issues relevant to new GPs. Deanery tutors deal with everyone else, encouraging professional education for established GPs, and practice-based education, for example. They work in close collaboration with PCTs, facilitating the PCT professional development agenda, and as such do a lot of advisory and organisational work rather than front-line education.

Summary

Postgraduate education in all its forms is fun, except perhaps for the poor dean who does not do any education or indeed professional practice any more. Trainers will always be needed, so opportunities are always there, and the personal rewards, if not the money, are tremendous. I would strongly recommend a career as a medical educationalist.

7

Is writing right for you?

Ruth Chambers

Writing can lead to all sorts of opportunities as a general practitioner (GP). You might have an academic leaning and use writing to disseminate the results of your research studies across the UK and beyond, leading to you presenting your work at conferences, or furthering your career as a researcher. You may find that you are regarded as a leading light in a special interest area having written in free-to-GP publications. You could come to be regarded as a champion of GPs if you use the GP weekly newspapers to air your views and move into medical journalism. You might write prose for your own satisfaction, or pen articles that are published for health service colleagues or patients to read. You could write information leaflets for patients or self-help materials — as paper or online resources. You might find that writing books gives you the greatest satisfaction, as 'how to books' for colleagues, erudite clinical texts or fiction for the general public.

If you like writing and others enjoy reading your work, you are likely to be versatile in the way you employ your talents and you might have a go at any or all of these possibilities. There are many openings for doctors who can write. Doctors have a head start as writers over people who graduate with English degrees or journalism qualifications — they have a specialty area to write about, human stories and a bank of interesting experiences.

Writing is never likely to be your main job as a doctor. You would lose the contact with patients or health service management that gives you the ideas and your writing could dry up. Also the money you receive for writing is likely to be disproportionately less than what you earn as a practising doctor, unless you are the very occasional doctor who writes a bestseller — of the kind that is turned into a Hollywood film, rather than a standard textbook.

Writing for academic or professional journals

If you are undertaking research, your writing may be more of a by-product of the research than the main activity. However, the writing up might be considered the most important part. If you spend years undertaking the actual research itself, disseminating the findings hangs on your expertise in writing the associated papers as much as the scientific design or outcomes. If you are the lead researcher you will probably be the main writer, but your co-authors should share the writing up and critique and improve your efforts.

Instead of reporting on your own research, you might write articles that report best practice, citing the published research of others. These might be discussion papers giving different perspectives when there are contrasting points of view, for example, about what interventions are most effective. You might have an idea for such an article, draft out a skeleton and phone or email the commissioning editor of your intended journal to see if they would be likely to accept such an article if you wrote it out in full.

You will be undertaking this type of writing for personal satisfaction or prestige, but not for money directly. Academics are judged by the number of papers that they have published, the quality of the journals that their papers are published in, as well as the nature and achievements of their research or educational work. In the long run, writing papers that are published in nationally and internationally acclaimed journals will help you to the top of your career and thus boost your income.

You could start by writing an editorial for a peer-reviewed or popular journal. These are often between 800–1200 words and written about a topical issue. You should have something new to say that is likely to be of interest to the target readers of that journal – or otherwise why would the editor want to publish it in the journal?

Another way for novice writers to start is to write up an interesting case, an unusual audit or a report of your achievements at work and submit it to a local or national journal, depending on how interesting it is. You should find a home for your piece if you pitch the article as the sort of material your chosen journal usually publishes and it is as interesting as you think.

Writing for medical newspapers

Writing for free-to-GP newspapers or similar publications for doctors, nurses or other health professionals does attract reasonable fees. Many such journals have a standard fee in the region of £150 to £200 per 1000–2000 words. Whether you consider this a good income depends on how quickly you write those words and if there are a series of revisions to make. Regular columnists or writers can probably write 1000-word articles in a couple of hours, whilst novices might take days writing and revising their article. A good tip for this style of writing is to aim your material at a GP who has been qualified for 10 years, and perhaps knows a great deal but needs updating. You need to develop a clear and simple style – sophisticated or complex prose would be out of place. The medical weeklies make their income from the advertisements they contain and you will need to be aware that your articles are commissioned to attract readers and indirectly to 'sell' advertising space.

You might start by mapping out one or more articles with an outline of key points. Look at the newspaper or publication for the name of the main editor, the features editor or clinical editor and email, phone or write directly. They will either commission you to write something or reject your ideas outright or ask for a revised outline. They may have something similar in the pipeline, so you should not be downhearted at such a rejection. Just develop a new angle, think about your presentation and try another newspaper or journal. Another way to start might be by joining up with someone who is already publishing regularly, and doing some joint articles so that you can learn the ropes, start to build your own reputation and attract commissions by yourself.

Your type of preferred writing might not be GP work-related articles, but something different like crosswords or descriptions of websites or pieces about cars, leisure or travel. Or you could write about your personal experiences in relation to your career for a publication like *BMJ Careers*.

Writing books

You are likely to be an established writer before you seriously consider writing a book. If you want to write a book in your professional area, the most obvious way is to approach a publisher that already produces books in your field for the readers whom you envisage buying your book. You will need to do some background research to find out what other competing books exist, perhaps by searching an online bookshop such as Amazon. You may need to study these potentially competitive books, by requesting them through your local library service, to determine if there really is a gap in the market which you can plug. If the market is overcrowded, switch your subject or angle.

Draw up a book proposal on your own or with colleagues, describing the contents, the target readership and the selling features of your suggested book. Submit it to one publisher at a time.[1] If the publisher is interested you will agree how royalties will be shared and the deadline for submitting your manuscript. Royalties are generally how most authors are paid, unless the authors are celebrities or have written previous best sellers for the general public, when they might get a payment up front that is deducted from royalties as they are accrued. It is well known that the income derived from royalties is relatively little when the length of time taken to write a book is taken into account. Generally, the authors or editors share a small proportion of the profits that the publishers make from a book once all the production, marketing and distribution costs have been deducted from sales. So, it is the satisfaction that comes from writing a book and seeing it read by others or used in their daily work that is important for an author of a book, rather than a monetary reward. Writing books gives an author prestige, which can boost their profile and enhance their career prospects or underpin other work-related activities such as providing consultancy.

If you are keen to write a book, but cannot find a publisher, another option open to you is self-publishing. It is possible to write a book and arrange for it to be published, so that you then market and sell your book, or pay for that service too. However, you are unlikely to have the marketing know-how or opportunities that a major publisher has, and you may find it difficult to sell your self-published book on a wide scale.

Another approach is to write one or more chapters in someone else's book, in the same way that this chapter has been written. Those editing the book or drawing up the book proposal might invite you to contribute because of your expertise or experience. In this case you will probably receive a nominal fee or equivalent in books from that publisher.

Writing for patients or the lay press

As well as the possibilities already described about writing articles or books for patients, you might try for a regular column in your local newspaper on health matters, or even be a regular columnist in a popular magazine. You might find an opening by contacting the publications directly with your ideas or finding a literary agent who can promote you.

You may be more interested in using your writing skills to produce patient information. You will need to be clear who it is for and if such information already exists — in which case use or refine that. Writing for patients will require you to work with some lay people to find out what they want to know, how detailed the information should be, what formats to use and how to present it in an appealing way so that the information is understandable.[2]

Advantages and disadvantages of writing as a GP career option

As with everything there are advantages and disadvantages to writing as well. Boxes 7.1 and 7.2 illustrate some of the more important points.

Box 7.1: Advantages of writing

- Disseminates your ideas far and wide – wonderful if you find it difficult to speak and command attention.
- Writing can be a passport to travel via conferences (even expenses are paid sometimes if you are a guest speaker).
- Writing is more or less within your control – few things about GP work are.
- Immense personal satisfaction using different skills other than medical ones, especially if unresolved longing for different career.
- Writing helps you think – it forces you to consider implications and be ahead of others' thinking.
- Writing overcomes hierarchies – as co-authors you are on an equal footing.
- Writing for GP press is generally well paid.
- Royalties from books are nice – you might regard them as outside your regular income and spend them on luxuries such as holidays or art.

Box 7.2: Disadvantages of writing

- Doesn't generally pay enough to live on – needs to be combined with GP work.
- Writers have to dedicate time to complete work – usually 'leisure' time.
- Writing is a solitary activity and can exclude family.

- People invite you to give presentations if you are published — requires different skills to writing and you may not have the skills or time.
- People expect you to give free advice to them, re-write their material.
- People who review your books are unnecessarily cruel to give them something to write about.
- Colleagues can be funny with you — publishing something is seen as implying you are an expert and you have to learn to weather snide remarks.

How to start

If you feel you have the urge to write then just write something, anything. But let it be about something you know about or want to tell others about. It could be a letter to the medical press or local newspaper. It could be an entry for a writing competition — a short piece on a set question or short story. It might be a report on some work you have been doing which you submit to the newspaper or journal likely to be appropriate for the type of piece it is. There is no point sending a chatty piece about your work that is not scientifically designed to an international journal, just because you think it interesting.

If you are unsure about the relevance of your work, check with the commissioning editor of the newspaper or publishing company (their phone or email addresses are usually given somewhere in the publication), or write a synopsis of your article or book and send it to the editor. Look for names and contact details in a current reference book.[1]

Go on a medical writing course, such as those run by Tim Albert Training (www.timalbert.co.uk). Find expert friends such as through the Society of Medical Writers (www.somw.org) or register at your local further education college or other body for a creative writing course.

It is unlikely that writing will become your sole career, but it can certainly become an integral part of your professional work or outside interests, that you combine with being a general practitioner to your great satisfaction.

References

1 *Writers' and Artists' Yearbook 2003* (2003) A and C Black, London.
2 Duman M (2003) *Producing Patient Information: how to research, develop and produce effective information resources.* King's Fund, London.

8

Working for a primary care trust

Peter Aquino, Bhupinder Kohli and
Claire Davidson

Primary care trusts (PCTs) are still fairly new in England and Wales. They were created by the Government in April 2000 and have the responsibility to develop and commission local health services in line with the health improvement programme. Although PCTs are primary care-based, they also work with secondary care doctors, to determine and commission how other health services are provided. As PCTs are local and autonomous organisations that have control of up to 80% of the local health budget, they should be better prepared than their larger health authority predecessors to meet the health needs of the population they serve.

Opportunities for clinicians

There are many opportunities for doctors wishing to work for a PCT, either as a member of the executive committee or as a clinical lead.

Executive committee

The executive committee is the backbone of a PCT and can have as many as nine health professionals (including up to five general practitioners (GPs)) from a total of 13 members. Other members include community consultants and health professionals allied to medicine, such as nurses, physiotherapists or occupational therapists, as well as some lay members.

GP members of the executive are selected from representative peer groups. If more GPs are selected than the number needed, then an election procedure will be instigated. Most executive members are highly motivated and want to make decisions that will have a positive impact on both health outcomes of patients and the working environment of local practices. An executive GP member may work up to four days a month and the executive chairperson around eight days a month. It is vital to negotiate with your own practice or employer on how to achieve a healthy balance between clinical and PCT work. There is a fixed yearly salary and additional locum reimbursement fee. Doctors may negotiate other working conditions depending on their commitment to their practice.

The remit of an executive member is interesting and variable. Primarily this entails ensuring that local primary care services are being developed, assessing local health needs, and identifying priority areas or problems that need to be addressed. Of course this is not a clinical role. Committee members spend their time at meetings discussing policy, reading discussion papers and networking with managers and other key members of the health and social care community, to develop policy and monitor implementation by the PCT. The currency is ideas and the tools are networking, communication skills and strategic management skills.

Clinical leads

Clinical leads are new posts for GPs, whose main task is to focus on the priority areas that have been identified by the PCT executive, such as diabetes, mental health or another key area that may be unique to that locality. Although the executive committee has overall responsibility for the operational management of the PCT, other demands mean that they do not have the time to dedicate to these key areas.

Clinical lead GPs are responsible for coordinating the development of services for the priority area. They help build links with the secondary sector, particularly with consultant clinicians in your specialised area. Other tasks include providing support and advice to local GPs on best practice, and ensuring that guidelines laid out in the national service framework (NSF) are being used locally and services are being developed accordingly. Some of their time will also be spent advising PCT staff and managers regarding their area of expertise. GPs who work as clinical leads work one to two sessions per week, and the pay and reimbursement is similar to the executive committee pro rata. The essential characteristics of a GP clinical lead are given in Box 8.1.

Box 8.1: Essential characteristics of a GP clinical lead

- Excellent communication skills.
- Good negotiation skills.
- Good timekeeping.
- Highly motivated.
- Worked in and familiar with the locality you wish to represent.
- Understand local and national health policies.
- In-depth knowledge and understanding of your priority area.

Points to consider

Do you have the time?

PCT work can be time-consuming as the job is demanding, so it is essential that you are able to balance time spent at your practice with time spent on PCT work. This can be tricky as invariably the two may clash occasionally. For example, you may have to do a home visit before a lunchtime PCT meeting or PCT meetings are arranged when you are scheduled for surgeries at the practice. You must also consider if it will affect your social or family commitments.

What will your practice say?

Your partners may have reservations about your PCT work. They may see it as creating an extra burden of work for them and possibly diverting your focus of attention away from the practice and day-to-day work with patients. They may be concerned about financial constraints as the reimbursement fee may not fully cover locum fees.

As happens often in life, people are suspicious of change; you must convince your partners that:

- you will still be focused on work with patients when at the practice, and this will always take priority
- there may be advantages in you working for the PCT as your partners will have easy access to you and so can readily raise any concerns they may have about PCT matters.

What area of expertise could you bring?

If you decide to work for the PCT, particularly in a clinical lead role, you must decide whether you have both the knowledge and the enthusiasm in your particular field. For example, if you think you would like to be the clinical lead for diabetes, ask yourself the following questions.

- Would my own partners consider me to be both enthusiastic and knowledgeable in the field of diabetes?
- Do you regularly see diabetic patients? If you do not run your practice's diabetes clinic then you should reconsider your decision to apply to work for a PCT.
- Are you able to discuss or debate with others at a high level and represent the needs of patients and clinicians – for example, discussing with the local member of parliament the problems that diabetic patients in your community face.

Do you possess the necessary characteristics?

You need to have all the essential characteristics listed in Box 8.1. If you lack a few, then your life will become increasingly difficult. For example, if you do not have good time management skills, this may ultimately lead to conflict with your practice, and if you lack enthusiasm, this may lead to boredom and low morale.

The advantages and disadvantages for taking on PCT work are listed in Box 8.2.

Box 8.2: Advantages and disadvantages of PCT work

Advantages
- Adds to your clinical interest.
- Personal experience and expertise can be shared.
- Opportunity to shape the future of local health services.
- Outcomes and quality of life for patients may be improved.

Disadvantages
- Can be time-consuming.
- Must negotiate with current employer for release from practice.
- Influence of a local practice can be variable.
- Possible lack of management support.
- Potential conflict within practice if colleagues have to cover practice.

Personal experience
Bhupinder Kohli

I am currently the chair of the professional executive committee (PEC) of Newham PCT, East London. I work in a socially deprived inner city area, and most of our local GPs were trained overseas and work single-handed or in small practices. The acute service providers struggle with the demands of the local population, who have some of worst health indices in the country.

PCT work has given me the opportunity to use my clinical knowledge to help influence management in a direction that is more locally sensitive and practical than central government dictates. For example, we have set up local incentive schemes for coronary heart disease and diabetes, which has improved the quality of care and helped to support underdeveloped practices. We have taken a multidisciplinary approach and have been able to support local practices, not only in clinical practice but also in providing premises and staff.

Through my work in the PCT I have been able to influence the best use of resources in commissioning for new services. It has given me the opportunity to work closely with consultants and local GPs. We are currently encouraging GPs to have a special interest in topics such as cardiology, gastroenterology (including using endoscopies), dermatology and rheumatology.

As PEC chair, I work two days per week for the PCT. I am often approached by local GPs and am happy to listen to their comments on local health. I do feel that working for a PCT makes a difference and I find the work satisfying and rewarding. Although I have been able to juggle PCT work and practice work, this has been difficult at times. As a clinician I can help individual patients in the consulting room but can benefit the wider population through my work with the PCT.

Personal experience

Claire Davidson

I was appointed as GP clinical lead for diabetes early last year, but my involvement in the development of our local diabetes services started several years ago. At that time approximately one-third of people with diabetes in Newham were receiving structured care from their GP surgery, but the participating GPs felt that they had no support from consultants, dietetic services or podiatry. Waiting times for diabetes outpatients' appointments were nine months or more, and a notable proportion of patients had no access to structured care. So my main remit was to ensure that primary care had the necessary support to provide diabetes services.

This involved lobbying managers and the members of the clinical board to fund a diabetes podiatrist, primary care dieticians and an auditor (to perform a baseline audit of diabetes care in general practice). From this we developed an incentive scheme, which is a structured way of providing administrative, educational, clinical and financial support to GPs. This extended into developing a 'model of care' with the local consultants and multidisciplinary team. After this work, we secured funding for additional posts, including a community diabetologist and additional diabetes specialist nurses, and some community projects, such as community diabetes health advocates and locality clinics.

Although at times the work is frustrating, onerous and poorly paid, it is extremely rewarding to feel that I am contributing to improving services for patients as well as ensuring that my colleagues receive the necessary support to deliver effective diabetes care.

Further information

www.doh.gov.uk/pct gives the Government's guidance on primary care trusts.

9

Flexible working in general practice

Petre Jones and Farzana Hussain

Flexibility is often thought of as working part-time. Well, often this is exactly what it means, but it also means trying to design jobs around people's individual needs rather than forcing people to work to predetermined patterns. This may mean working part-time, or working at different times to work around particular issues, which should be particularly possible in general practice given the relatively small teams in which we work. In this chapter we will look at some of the issues and in particular use The Project Surgery in East London as an example of some ways in which it can be done. We have tried to separate flexible working and childcare issues from women's issues because, although these are the main hurdles facing women in their careers, increasingly men are taking a bigger role in childcare and, particularly through illness, may well have a need for flexible working. These are not issues for only women to think about.

There are many reasons why people should want to work 'flexibly'. Childcare is the commonest, but illness and family issues are also important reasons, and some of us of course do have significant lives to lead outside medicine. In terms of recruitment and retention an increase in flexible working is vital.

The Department of Health in the white paper *Improving Working Lives* emphasised the need for flexible, meaning part-time, training and careers as well as other ways of making life in the NHS better for the workforce.[1] It gives lots of examples, but very few in primary care.

Deanery mediated flexibility

The flexible training scheme is run by the deaneries and provides full daytime funding for training grades to work part-time, with a minimum commitment of 50%. Contact the flexible training dean at your deanery for more details. Usually trusts jump at the chance to have an extra person on the team who is virtually free to them. However, I have known a trust decline on the grounds that to train you need some out-of-hours experience, and the deanery funds will not cover this. Thus there may be a small cost to the trust, but most are enlightened enough to get over this. This scheme would help someone training for general practice, through the senior house officer (SHO) years, but stops when you become a general practice registrar (GPR).

GPR posts can also be made fairly flexible, in terms of part-time, and, as all GPRs are in reality supernumerary, most training practices will be able to work the GPR's job around any needs that they have, as long as this does not compromise training. For a full-time GPR to become part-time they simply need to agree this with their trainer and the number of sessions can be reduced with the rate of pay being reduced pro rata and the training period lengthened, again pro rata, by simple arithmetic.

Once trained the deanery can still offer some flexible and part-time options. The flexible career scheme is designed to fund people to work up to an average of 50% time, but the sessions do not have to be fixed each week, as long as on average they add up to the contracted total. Thus someone with children might work more in term time and less in holiday time, or someone with a recurrent illness might work more when well and then cut down when ill.

The retainer scheme was originally set up to help women with childcare commitments to work part-time in general practice and retain their skills. A retainer can work up to four sessions in general practice, in a practice that has been approved by the deanery, and they will have part funding for their work.

The returner scheme is another way of helping GPs with different career paths. It provides refresher training funded by the deanery to people who for example may be returning to work after a few years break due to illness.

Flexibility in practice

How can practices help their staff by working around their other commitments? One might expect that practices as small organisations could work out all sorts of ways of being flexible, particularly as the personal medical services (PMS) and general medical services (GMS) contracts recognise the part-timer varying from 25% to 75% time, and allow for out-of-hours opt-outs. There are certainly part-time options available, as principals and in salaried posts, but problems in getting cover and traditional working practices often prevent these from becoming more than just part-time and truly flexible. Often too the imagination or the motivation is lacking. Interestingly, *Improving Working Lives*[1] has very little to offer GPs in practice beyond the training grades, particularly for GP principals, so it is up to us to make it happen.

The Project Surgery as an example of truly flexible working

We both work in The Project Surgery in East London, and here are some of the ways we have found to be flexible around Petre's recurring illness and Farzana's childcare issues.

We have almost 3000 patients, to whom we provide a patient-centred primary care service. We have 1.75 whole time equivalent (wte) partners, 1.7 GPRs, 1 practice nurse, a half-time cognitive behavioural therapy (CBT) therapist, and sessional men's health nurse, benefits adviser, asylum seekers adviser, community psychiatric nurse (CPN), and attached district nurse and health visitor and an art and a gardening project. So much for the traditional care!

Flexibility for the staff

We have tried to identify staff personal needs through an open discussion policy and through appraisal.

For reception staff, needs have been about fitting working hours around family commitments and being able to take time off to take family to hospital, etc. Other key staff needs have been about understanding inexperience and supported learning, being aware of and supported through illness, and understanding personal fears.

For Farzana, it is about flexible hours when she is tired from pregnancy, making time for antenatal appointments, etc., recognising and supporting her professional learning needs and, above all, childcare. She felt uncomfortable leaving either of her babies with a childminder or nursery and her working hours would have made this difficult anyway. So, instead, we adapted the surgery staff room a little and found a nanny who comes in when Farzana is doing surgery to look after the children. At other times the whole team just chip in and look after them as required and, surprisingly perhaps, this is not really disruptive and is certainly good for team morale. Above all the arrangement is very flexible.

The strengths of our flexible working and in-house childcare arrangements for Farzana are as follows.

- Maternity leave was shortened on both occasions! Farzana came back to work after each child at her own pace and did not have to worry about arranging childcare. A gradual return to work would be hard to arrange as regards childcare. With our system the childcare was there when she needed it for as many sessions as she needed. Farzana felt that six months was too long to be away from the surgery, and certainly the surgery benefits hugely by having both partners around.
- One common parental fear is what will the carer do when they reach the end of their tether. Farzana had the security of knowing that all the team members, as well as the nanny, are happy to chip

in and look after the children as needed, so no one gets too fraught. For example, when little baby Zarina is being fed, 'big' brother Usmaan can get a bit jealous and upset, so our secretary might take Usmaan out with her to the post office to get some office supplies. Or if Usmaan is getting restless, 30 minutes at the reception desk or watching our practice manager will often send him to sleep.

- Particularly when Zarina was very small it was comforting for Mum to know that she was just upstairs and Mum could nip up and check on her in between patients if necessary.
- Farzana feels in control of her children's care.

This arrangement would not work without a huge amount of team-work and real affection for the children from all the staff, and in return the practice team works more closely together, sharing non-work-related skills and experience, as if this were an ongoing team-building exercise. Without this affection and desire to care, the system simply would not work.

Flexibility is also important to deal with Petre's illness. Petre suffers from a recurrent depressive illness. He is on long-term medication and has had quite a variety of talking therapies. He has had three past hospital admissions and has regular psychiatric follow-up. He has a tendency to overwork to boost low self-esteem.

To help with these needs his workload is carefully regulated. He has time specifically set aside for management tasks, for teaching and 'down' time; one day every two weeks when he comes into work, he usually catches up a bit, or paints, or goes for a run. He finds time for at least two runs per week and we have fitted a shower to deal with this. Running is a good way for him to relax, clear his head, think and recharge. Farzana, and indeed all the team, keep an eye out for him being stressed and are all willing to listen if he has had a tough patient for example. He gets time out for appointments, including psychotherapy, and our men's health nurse practises her phlebotomy skills to check his lithium levels. Finally, in our business plan, and now almost in reality, we were to build up a contingency fund of £20k to fund the costs of locums, and admission to his psychiatrist's private unit, in the event of another recurrence, so as to reduce the negative impact of the illness with a rapid high-quality admission to hospital under someone he knows and trusts.

These are some of the practical flexibilities we have developed so far, and they arise from our partnership culture. They also depend on close trust and teamwork within the practice. We have worked hard to build this in the following ways.

- All staff person specifications used at recruitment include an essential skill of being able to be supportive of colleagues within a team, and we took this seriously at interview.
- We had our training and team-building week before we opened (we have been running for one year) to get the team working together, using group building skills learned in the process of course organising.
- The partnership buys food for lunch time, so the whole team can meet up in the staff room and share lunch, and childcare.
- We go out for practice evenings about once every month.
- We run monthly staff meetings which are informal and either look at clinical governance and the way the practice works or our practice education programme.
- We hold regular formal and informal debrief and supervision sessions.

We have just become a PMS practice and one of our aims as set out in our application form is to aid recruitment and retention by adopting employment policies and practices which aim to support individual staff needs.

Obviously we have been very fortunate at The Project Surgery but I believe there are lessons here for every practice if they want to be more flexible.

- It starts with the partners and the partnership culture. A couple of away days or some facilitated meetings might explore the issues for the partnership, and make it clear if this is a way forward for them.
- Building teams is important. We have a team of about eight core people, the perfect size for group functioning. Perhaps a larger practice could break down into two or three 'practice' units, or job-based teams.
- Spend time, energy and money on the team – joint training, time together, food!

- Be imaginative in your solutions. Farzana is very good at coming up with unusual ideas, which Petre then turns into real solutions. Neither of us worries particularly about how things are usually done. The childcare arrangements started as a wacky idea which we did not think could be done, until we looked in detail at how we would do it. This is the beauty of a partnership. One can do things in ways to suit the partners, within the law of course.

Childcare

Until we sat down to write this neither of us, with seven children between us, had heard of the NHS Childcare Strategy, which arose out of *Improving Working Lives*.[1] Following on from the national strategy, each area should apparently have a local strategy, and a childcare coordinator who can point parents in the right direction for suitable childcare.

Workplace nurseries

Local strategies are supposed to take GP issues into account, and should include plans for workplace nurseries. Of course unless the GP works from a hospital site it is very unlikely that the nursery will be at the GP's workplace. There are practices with workplace nurseries, however, arising out of recognition that childcare is a major issue for many GPs. Having the space will be a problem for many practices, but there is the huge advantage that with a workplace nursery, child-care costs suddenly attract tax relief for a partner, making them much cheaper. In The Project Surgery, as mentioned above, we have moved beyond the adjacent nursery to having our small children cared for in the practice by an employed nanny and, when needed, members of the practice team.

Traditional childcare solutions

- Family.
- Nanny – unregulated and provides care in your home.
- Childminder – must be a registered childminder if they provide paid childcare for more than two hours. In its own unique way

Ofsted is trying its best to overregulate and reduce the morale of childminders.

- Au pairs, whose main role is to learn a new language, provide unregulated childcare, as a subsidiary role.

How rights differ in general practice depending on the contract

Different contractual arrangements for GPs bring different employment rights relating to childcare. The following are examples of the different rights different GPs can expect for emergency childcare:

- PCT employed salaried GP – entitled to six days emergency childcare
- practice employed salaried GP – no entitlement to emergency childcare
- GP principal, PMS or GMS – no rights and very little support.

One could say the same about paternity leave, for example, and it usually boils down to the GP principal getting the worst deal, although some practice salaried jobs in the past have been dreadful.

However, this does not have to be the case. It ought to be possible for us all to enjoy the terms and conditions of the best. For example, in 1992 Petre and one of his then partners were both off work on paternity leave, for one month each. The then Family Health Service Authority (FHSA) even reimbursed some of the locum fees from the time when their paternity leave overlapped. This was all because of a well written partnership deed, a lot of which is about good will and imagination.

A pot-pourri of money issues

- Obviously working part-time you will earn less, but a part-timer in a high earning practice could still earn more than a full-timer in a low earning practice.
- Remember that you might be able to claim working families' tax credit or childcare tax credit (which covers some of the costs of childcare).

- Get locum expense insurance for GP principals and get long-term income protection insurance for everyone, so that if you become too unwell to work you will still have an income to support your-self and your dependants.

Women GPs

First the value-laden stereotypes. Women GPs prefer to work part-time, do lots of family planning, psychiatry and child health and are perceived by patients as being more empathetic than men.

With that out of the way, we will consider some facts. There are still more male than female principals, although women outnumber men as GPRs. Part-timers are seven times more likely to be women, but full-time women still outnumber part-timers 2 to 1 (RCGP Information Sheet).[2] It is also true that when asked about areas of lead responsibility within the practice it was only in women's health and antenatal work that more women than men took lead respon-sibility. Computers, finance, minor surgery, meeting external visitors and annual reporting were all dominated by men. What is less clear is whether this is about patient choice, practice partners' choice or women GPs' choice. As to empathy, that is surely not the preserve of one gender.

It seems that the two things that are most problematic for GPs are childcare and the need for flexible working, both touched on above.

Maternity and other rights

- An employed women is entitled to 26 weeks paid maternity leave and if employed for 26 weeks by the twenty-sixth week of pregnancy can take a further 26 weeks additional maternity leave which is usually unpaid.
- Maternity leave can start from week 29.
- Women principals are eligible to receive maternity locum reim-bursements for 26 weeks, but this does not of course guarantee getting a locum.
- You cannot work at all whilst on maternity leave.
- New parents who are employed are entitled to ask, and have re-quests taken seriously, for flexible working, i.e. changes in working

times, changes to the total hours worked and the opportunity to work from home where possible.

- A new father with six months employment can claim up to two consecutive weeks paternity leave and statutory paternity pay.
- A new adoptive parent can claim 26 weeks adoptive leave and statutory adoptive pay.
- A mother or father can claim 13 weeks unpaid parental leave up to the child's fifth birthday, or eighteenth birthday if disabled or adopted.

Does gender discrimination exist in medicine?

A report by the Royal College of Physicians of London in 2001, chaired by Professor Carol Black, looked at why there were so few women compared to men in academic and senior grades in general medicine and associated specialties. Their conclusions were that more needed to be done to meet the needs of women for childcare and flexible working. We now have a range of flexible options and childcare options arising from *Improving Working Lives.*[1]

However, flexible training opportunities are limited and flexible career options even more so. The National Childcare Strategy remains largely unimplemented and, even if it were, the options of childminding, nurseries and nannies are not always available, suitable or of an appropriate quality. Nurseries are never likely to be based in many practices. As long as this situation continues there will always be organisational issues which discriminate against women on the basis of their gender and role in raising families.

What of individual attitudes? The health service is full of people, and for everyone who feels more should be done to support working parents, there will be someone who feels this is just putting work on to other people and that is unfair. Beyond this there will, as with any group of fallible humans, always be the odd ones who 'think' in gender discriminatory ways. The following are some real examples.

- A pregnant woman GP who is dehydrated from hyperemesis and urinary tract infections should just work through the pregnancy regardless of the fact that she can barely stand up. Male partners who are ill get time off.

- The other (male) partners can make major decisions about the future of the partnership without even talking to the female partner.
- When working at the GP Co-operative alongside a senior (male) GP, the female GP finds him repeatedly questioning her decisions and talking down to her.

Yes, unfair discrimination does exist, and we should work against it, but this is only a reflection of humankind as a whole.

Tips on being a woman GP

- If you need a chocolate break, stop and buy that KitKat and take five minutes for yourself.
- Be flexible with colleagues who need favours, because you will be asking for favours in return.
- Children go to birthday parties, so have a box of suitable presents ready bought. You do not want to have to make special shopping trips.
- If you need to be around at the surgery at the end of the day, feed and change the baby before you go home so when you get in you can put the baby down and have five minutes to relax before being on duty as a mum again.
- Accept every offer of help.
- It's good enough to be 'good enough'. Do not try to be the perfect mother or the perfect GP.

Summary

Our purpose in writing this chapter has been to show what can and what could be done to increase flexibility and create imaginative childcare solutions. If this were done we would retain more of those doctors, particularly women, who currently get to SHO grades and then leave medicine or fail to work to their full potential. We cannot afford to miss out on their talents any longer.

References

1　Department of Health (1999) *Improving Working Lives*. DoH, London.
2　RCGP (1998) *Women General Practitioners*. RCGP Information Sheet 14. Royal College of General Practitioners, London.

10

Assorted hobbies

Petre Jones

One of the great joys of general practice is that it offers you many chances to explore your interests, without leaving the skilled and interesting field you trained for. Previous chapters have looked at some of these, but in this chapter I want to look at some of the variety of opportunities which are on offer.

Secondary type care

There is nothing new about GPs doing some secondary care. GPs in this country have always been to some extent involved in hospital-type care and in countries such as Nigeria and India virtually all GPs do secondary care, although in these healthcare systems the general practice is not quite the same as we would recognise here. Opportunities include the clinical assistant post, hospital practitioner grades, 'GPs with a special interest' and a variety of informal arrangements.

The key issues with all these options are:

- Where will you do it?
- What sort of work would you do?
- Who will pay you and how much?
- What training will you need?
- To whom, if anyone, will you be responsible?

Where will you do it?

This is an odd first question perhaps, but what you do and how tends to flow from where you do your work. So, with the old style clinical assistant posts and hospital practitioner grades, GPs work in hospital as part of hospital teams and they are responsible to consultants and managed by hospital managers. Clinical assistants usually do not require much additional training beyond the vocational training scheme (VTS) and do more or less senior house officer (SHO) level stuff. Hospital practitioners tend to work to a higher level but require a bit more specialist training. Gynaecology, rheumatology, general medical outpatients services and ophthalmology etc. all offer these posts.

In contrast GPs with a special interest work in primary care, usually running specialist clinics in the practice, providing what would normally be considered secondary care. In these services the GP is the boss, and in control of the whole thing, but will also often need quite extensive specific training.

Clinics where access to technology is not very important include:

- dermatology
- drug abuse
- headaches
- rheumatology
- psychosexual counselling.

Clinics in primary care with some investment include:

- minor general surgery
- endoscopy
- minor ophthalmic surgery.

Areas less suitable for the GP with a special interest, because of a need for on-site technology, because there are not usually long waits or because multidisciplinary teams are needed include:

- orthopaedics — obviously would not work without x-ray
- paediatrics — usually does not have long waiting times
- care of the elderly or community psychiatry — need teams.

Who will pay you and how much?

The hospital appointments are advertised by the trusts who fund the post. There is no training element to the funding from deaneries, unlike the 50/50 funded SHO posts, so there is no training requirement. Pay rates are nationally negotiated and relatively low. You can find them set out in the medical financial press.

For the community-based special interest clinic, things are different. These are funded by primary care organisation (PCO) commissioners. Funds for expensive secondary care referrals to specialties with long waiting lists are diverted to pay specialist GPs to do some of the work, with the GP negotiating the cost for each case based on professional time and practice overhead costs. So, in Newham in East London, long waiting lists for neurology were made up largely by referrals for headache. Setting up a headaches clinic, run by a GP who had been a medical registrar, meant cutting the waiting lists and was a more rational use of resources.

What training will you need?

For clinical assistantships you will need very little extra training, but for all the other options you will need extensive training, which is not surprising as GP training equips you to be a GP not a specialist. Herein lies the biggest drawback with the specialist GP, particularly for those of us who did GP training early in our careers because we wanted to be GPs.

However, many GPs have previously enjoyed specialist careers. Understandably having gained skills you will be keen to use them. So, for example, with a career to specialist registrar level in general surgery before starting general practice you might be interested in running a primary care surgical service. As long as your past training can be brought to bear on an area where commissioners might want to deal with long waiting lists, and technology does not limit you, you could investigate setting up such a service.

Those without skills already will need to undertake quite extensive further training, perhaps passing one of the various college diplomas. The training can be tailor-made for your needs.

Having trained for your new service you will need to get accredited by the PCO before the commissioners will agree to set up a contract with you and start to pay you for your work. They will want to make sure that the practice, the premises and the equipment are of a suitable standard to provide your service. As part of that accreditation process they may want to see your training accredited with an independent diploma or qualification. You may have this already, or membership of a specialist college, but it seems now there is a diploma to meet most occasions. Examples are as follows:

- screening clinic for returning travellers – Royal College of Physicians (RCP) Diploma in Tropical Medicine
- drug abuse service – RCGP Certificate in Management of Drug Abuse
- dermatology clinic – King's College London, Diploma in Dermatology
- rheumatology clinic – Bath University, Diploma in Primary Care Rheumatology
- psychosexual clinic – Lancaster University, Diploma in Psychosexual Counselling.

However, never confuse getting a diploma with acquiring competence. You need to be clinically competent in any role you undertake and a diploma does not prove this. Nor does a lack of a diploma say anything negative about you. Sadly, commissioning PCOs may not understand this point of view as the diploma seems a convenient quality end-point to measure.

Reservations

Personally I have some questions about all this.

- The way we approach people in primary care and the clinical skills we use are different from secondary care. Very few practitioners can be expected to be able to maintain skills in both approaches. GPs may become less patient-centred, whilst as a specialist they may use the 'physical, psychological and social' diagnostic technique of the GP and lose the 'cast the net wide within the physical domain' approach of the physician for example, to the detriment of both sectors.

- General practice is vast, with many areas for improvement. Should we not get our own house in order before we extend to sorting out secondary care?
- Lots of GPs doing extra work in the relative isolation of specialist clinics raises the question of keeping up to date and to standard.
- More fundamentally, I worry about the direction that this might take general practice. As GPs we are so much more than the sum of the specialties that our work touches. Specialist GPs move us closer to a polyclinic approach where the patient tends to be reduced to different illness elements. The general practice I trained for and teach is about holistic care and continuity. It is about seeing a patient with an acute peptic ulcer and remembering his past depression and very low self-esteem and realising that by allowing him to make choices about his ulcer he will be empowered and will make one more step along his pathway to valuing himself and reducing the risk of self-harm. It is about knowing a family and knowing how the matriarchal grandmother finds it hard to admit to the stressed daughter that her angina is worse, but will tell you because you stayed calm when the asthmatic grandchild had a bad attack. I worry about specialisms in general practice because I care about holistic care.

Other interests and activities

There is a vast range of interests and activities undertaken by GPs, and we can only really give a taste of some of the opportunities. Most of the types of work in this section are not usually undertaken by doctors newly out of VTS. It is usually GPs who have spent a few years establishing their GP credentials who then branch out into new areas, sometimes as a new challenge and sometimes to refresh their career. One might undertake a new role for a few years and then perhaps move on. One's own career can be as varied as the nature of general practice itself. Here are some examples, in no particular order.

British Association of Immediate Care Doctors

Members of the British Association of Immediate Care Doctors (BASICS) provide immediate and pre-hospital care in emergencies, from the everyday car crash to major disasters such as the Clapham rail crash. BASICS is a charity and the doctors' time and equipment costs are underfunded, and of course making oneself available to be called by the ambulance service to the scene of an incident can be very disruptive to routine primary care. However, this is truly life-saving work. Training is available leading to a Certificate of Pre-hospital Care or a Diploma in Immediate Care, from Edinburgh University.

Forensic medical examiner

Police surgeons look after people in custody, and the work is not as glamorous as the television portrayals. They attend police stations at the request of custody sergeants to provide healthcare to people who may be drunk, drugged, mentally ill or just an asthmatic needing an inhaler. They also are frequently asked to appear as witnesses in court. This is another varied role that is frequently disruptive to practice life, but at least this one is reasonably paid. There is a MSc and Diploma in Forensic Medicine run by the University of Edinburgh.

Another forensic medical examiner role that is more circumscribed is that of doing specialist examinations on victims of rape or sexual abuse. This is fascinating, important and grim.

Prison Medical Service

The Prison Medical Service has recently been removed from the Home Office and placed firmly within the remit of the NHS, with each prison being associated with a PCO and undertaking clinical governance, etc. There are a number of openings for GPs to work with the service and they are very keen to recruit. The work ranges from routine medical screening of new inmates with the help of screening nurses, to challenging work with inmates. A lot of the work is acute psychiatry, with a high number of people with psychosis, behavioural problems and depression, with self-harm prevention and suicide prevention a key element. Substance misuse, drugs and alcohol accounts for another large chunk of the work, and then there is the 'physical' illness, which can be anything from tuberculosis to heart disease, to injuries and long-term disabilities. And, yes, there is a Diploma in Prison Medicine, based at the University of Nottingham.

Occupational health

Occupational health (OH) is a whole specialty in its own right and many large employers will have a substantial OH department or contract out to one. However, there are opportunities for GPs to work within an OH department and for smaller firms to provide a full OH service, backed up by OH nurses. The role includes health assessments, the effect of health and disability on work, and the effects of work on health. Again a diploma exists for those who want it – the Diploma in Occupational Health of the Faculty of Occupational Medicine, RCP, London.

Sports medicine

Like occupational health this can range from doing the odd session for a local sports club, through being a premiership team doctor, right up to running a full-time sports clinic service, which is rapidly becoming its own sub-specialty. Again there is the inevitable diploma to work for, the Diploma in Sports Medicine, Royal College of Surgeons (RCS), Edinburgh. One big advantage is that you are able to see all the home games! Local hospital sports clinics also exist, which may be interested in appointing clinical assistants and hospital practitioners.

Benefits Agency work

Someone has to do the medicals for all work tests, appeals and attendance allowance and disability living allowance (DLA). Traditionally, older doctors have done this work after retirement, but there are opportunities for others. Try as I might I just cannot make this sound interesting, sorry Benefits Agency!

Insurance medicals

All GP principals are familiar with doing medical attendance reports and insurance medicals. Well, if you really want to, there is a market for doctors to do extra insurance work, where for example the applicant has no GP or the GP has not known them very long. Directories of doctors willing to do this work exist, but once you have let a few insurance companies know you are interested in this type of work, and proved yourself to be reliable and efficient, you should get a nice stream of work, and extra income.

Private sector GPs

There are not a lot of private GPs around, but there are some, particularly in large cities. They tend to focus on medical examinations for work and insurance, and private health assessments. Some work as retainers in large hotels, so that when a guest is ill the doctor can be called without too much fuss about who to contact. Another area of private work is the cosmetic market. I know of no GPs who are also consultant aesthetic plastic surgeons, but there are opportunities for GPs to be trained in botulinum toxin injections and laser tattoo removal. Capital costs for this work are high if you set up your own service, but you might well find work in an existing clinic.

Voluntary sector work

There are a huge range of opportunities here, but they are not high earners. I know of doctors running clinic services in homeless persons shelters, usually at a very important but basic level, because of the problems of funding medication for example. I work for two fostering agencies as medical adviser, screening applicants' medical assessment forms and attending about six panel meetings per year to discuss the selection of prospective foster carers. Working with social workers and foster carers is different and fascinating, and gives me new insights into people and how they think and work. I have also on occasion been asked to run first aid courses for youth organisations, and run discussions on health issues. One could give more examples, but the point is that there is plenty to do if you want to.

Enhanced services

Before we end this chapter, remember that the general medical services (GMS) and personal medical services (PMS) contracts allow ordinary GPs to provide a range of optional enhanced services within their practices that will be reimbursed by the PCO. There are nationally agreed enhanced services such as anticoagulant clinics, drug abuse services, intrauterine device (IUD) fitting services, and sexual health services and the possibility of locally agreed enhanced services. All of these are designed to fit within the usual boundaries of general practice so will not require extensive extra training, but are essentially within our existing job and title deeds. It is up to you to decide if these are extending your career or are part of your usual service.

Diplomatosis

Having mentioned a host of diplomas in this section, it is worth saying a few words about acquiring diplomas. In my course organiser role I am often asked which of the college diplomas are important for someone's career. My answer is simple. Membership of the Royal College of General Practitioners (MRCGP) is important, the rest are not.

MRCGP is now mandatory for anyone interested in training or education, and in many places is considered important in getting a partnership job. To that end, and considering the rate of brain cell death, I suggest people start sitting the modules towards the end of the GPR year, although one can always do membership by assessment later.

Of all the other diplomas around that people tend to pick up as they pass through SHO jobs, I have never found any that make much difference to anyone. You will need a family planning certificate if you want to work in family planning clinics, but it is not necessary for doing contraception work in general practice. You will need an IUD Certificate of Competence if you want to teach IUD fitting in a family planning clinic, but apart from those, Diploma of Child Health (DCH), Diploma of Geriatric Medicine (DGM), Diploma of the Royal College of Obstetrics and Gynaecology (DRCOG), etc. are not important to general practice. The most important thing is to be well trained and above all competent, and the examinations prove neither, and honestly they are not going to get a job for you.

Having said all that, they do have some value for some people. Most of us are what is called activist learners; we learn by doing, by being involved and gaining experience, which we can then draw on when we need to reflect and do book work. If this is you, I suggest you keep a log of anything interesting you did not know that comes up in the day's work and read about it later. If you do this you will learn what you need to know.

However, some people learn in a different way; they are the reflectors who take it all in first before feeling they can make decisions. For these people book learning may well come first, so they have a good background knowledge before tackling a problem.

These people might do well to buy a good text book before each SHO job, read it through and then apply it to the situations they meet. If this describes you then you may learn a lot from the study involved in working for a diploma, and for you it may be worthwhile to do some diplomas purely to stimulate your learning.

The only other valid reason for doing a diploma that I can see is if an outside body wants it as a shorthand way of saying you are competent to do something you wish to do. This is a rather lazy way for agencies to assess competence, as there is all the difference in the world between passing an exam, however well designed, and providing a competent clinical service day to day, but they do have to base their decisions on something, and this is the main justification for the vast range of rather specialised diplomas I have mentioned.

I did the DGM many years ago because I did a care of the elderly job followed by a psychiatry of the elderly job. I enjoyed it, and the clinical exam was interesting, but as to my career, well it has only been commented on once in the last 15 years. An MDU lawyer asked me if it meant I was particularly more interested in elderly people, and I had to truthfully answer 'No', and no one has asked about it before or since.

Final thoughts

During the course of this book we have looked at general practice working arrangements in all their breadth. Our specialty is unique in that it can be undertaken in many different ways and with so many subdivisions of interest. There is however another aspect of the breadth of general practice work which we have not considered.

Recently a colleague of mine in another practice was suddenly taken ill. This left the practice with a manpower problem at very short notice. Of course, as one does – or should do – my partner and I offered to cover a couple of the sessions to help out in a crisis.

In my practice, in inner city Newham, most of the patients are under 50 years old, with richly mixed ethnicity. The common health issues are mental illness, somatisation disorders, asthma and complex social problems. I find this fascinating. When I went to my friend's practice, again in Newham, I had a surgery in which nearly all of the patients were ethnically Bengali, over 50 years old and suffering from raised blood pressure, diabetes Type 2, or ischaemic heart disease, or most often all three. It was such a breath of fresh air to deal with general medical problems in older people, and deal with just one ethnic group.

Two practices so close together and, on paper, very similar to each other have totally different populations and therefore totally different types of work to be done. I am toying with the idea of doing the odd session at my friend's practice just for the experience and to brush up my skills.

You will never discover these sorts of differences by simply thinking about contractual arrangements, however important these are. This underlines the huge variety of work there is that is open to the GP, and this variety is not surprising when one considers the huge range of people that we serve.

And so to the very heart of what general practice is. In all the changes that have been inflicted on us by our well-meaning masters, with templates and quality markers, new contracts and 'advanced' access, the central point of it all is the moment when doctor and patient meet in the consultation. Two fallible human beings – one with a set of expert skills and knowledge, the other vulnerable with a health concern they want to deal with – meet and interact in a way that touches both, leaving the healing role validated and the patient hopefully strengthened. OK, I admit this is a rather romanticised view and not many consultations attain this idyll, but the point for me is that in all we do there is nothing more important than the consultation, and we serve our patients and our careers best if we remember never to take this for granted.

As to jobs and contracts, we are in a time when we can all have career paths as varied as we choose. Already portfolio careers are with us, and during your career you will have endless new opportunities to earn, do something different, and have fun. I hope you enjoy your career path as much as I am enjoying mine, and retain your love of meeting patients.

Petre Jones
May 2004

Index

academic general practice 63–9
  Clinical Academic Careers in the UK
      64
  PCTs 66
  personal experiences 68–9
  practice-based teaching 65–8
  research 66–8
  salaried GPs 66
  university-based 64–5
academic journals, writing 82–3
accounts/accountants
  financial issues 40
  partnerships 44–5
administrators, practice 28–9
adoption leave 36
annual leave 34

balance, income/workload/patient
    care 4–9
banking policy, partnerships 45

BASICS *see* British Association of
    Immediate Care Doctors
behaviour, partnerships 16–23
Belbin's group roles, partnerships
      17–18
benefits agency work 115
books, writing 84–5
British Association of Immediate Care
    Doctors (BASICS) 114

child care, general practice 103–4
Clinical Academic Careers in the UK
      64
clinical governance 4
clinical leads, PCTs 90–1
compassionate leave 35
compatibility issues, partnerships
      5–9
compulsory expulsion, Partnership
    Deeds 33

conflict resolution, partnerships   18, 19
contingency   3
contracts, locums   56, 57–8
culture, partnerships   13–16

deanery mediated flexibility   98–9
decision-making
    formal   26–7
    joint   25–6
democracy and shared responsibility, partnership model   24
diplomatosis   117–18
discrimination, general practice   106–7
dynamics, partnerships   16–23

enhanced services   117
ethos, partnerships   13–16
executive committee, PCTs   90
executive partner system, partnership model   23–4, 27
expenses, pooling   42–3
expulsion, Partnership Deeds   33

financial issues
    accountants   40
    expenses, pooling   42–3
    good will   43–5
    outside income   41–2
    partnerships   39–45
    pooling income   40–1
    shares   39–40
    tax   39–40
    see also income; money
flexibility
    deanery mediated   98–9
    examples   99–103
    general practice   97–108
    locums   55–6
    in practice   99
    premises   37
    Project Surgery   99–103
    salaried GPs   49, 52
    work   2–3
forensic medical examiners   114

formal decision-making   26–7
formal models, partnerships   23–31
fox, conflict mode style   19

general practice
    child care   103–4
    discrimination   106–7
    flexibility   97–108
    maternity leave   100, 105–6
    money   104–5
    paternity leave   105–6
    personal needs   100–4
    women GPs   105–7
general practice senior registrars (GPSRs), salaried GPs   51
'good enough'   3–4, 107
good will, financial issues   43–5
GPSRs see general practice senior registrars
groupthink, partnerships   14, 15–16

higher professional education (HPE) directors, postgraduate education   78–9
hobbies   109–18
    BASICS   114
    benefits agency work   115
    diplomatosis   117–18
    enhanced services   117
    forensic medical examiners   114
    insurance medicals   116
    occupational health (OH)   115
    Prison Medical Service   114–15
    private sector GPs   116
    secondary type care   109–13
    sports medicine   115
    voluntary sector work   116
holidays see leave arrangements
HPE directors see higher professional education directors

Improving Working Lives   103, 106
income
    balance   4–9
    outside   41–2

pooling   40–1
see also financial issues; money
income protection insurance   2
The Inner Apprentice   6–8
insurance, income protection   2
insurance medicals   116
IT (information technology),
    locums   58–9

job applications, salaried GPs   51–2
job security, locums   59–60
job sharing   30
joining the practice, Partnership
    Deeds   32–3
joint decision-making, partnership
    model   25–6

larger practices, partnerships
    18–20
lay press, writing for   85
leasing premises   38
leave arrangements
    locums   57
    Partnership Deeds   34–6
leaving the practice, Partnership
    Deeds   32–4
legal issues
    joint decision-making   26
    Partnership Deeds   11–13, 32–45
linking practices   20–1
locums   55–61
    advantages   55–7
    contracts   56, 57–8
    disadvantages   57–60
    flexibility   55–6
    IT   58–9
    job security   59–60
    leave arrangements   57
    NI   58
    parking   59
    pay   56, 57, 58, 60
    tax   58, 60

management team, partnership
    model   25
managers, practice   28–9

maternity leave   35
    general practice   100, 105–6
maternity pay, salaried GPs   49, 52
medical newspapers, writing   83–4
money   4
    general practice   104–5
    see also financial issues; income
moral stances, partnerships   13–15
mutual assessment periods,
    Partnership Deeds   32–3

National Insurance (NI), locums   58
Neighbour, Roger   6–8, 12–13
NI *see* National Insurance
non-judgemental value rating scales
    (NJVRS)   68, 12–13
notes summarisers, postgraduate
    education   76
number of partners, partnerships
    18–23

occupational health (OH)   115
outside income   41–2
owl, conflict mode style   19
owning premises   36–7

parking, locums   59
part-time working   30
Partnership Deeds   11–13, 32–45
    compulsory expulsion   33
    expulsion   33
    joining the practice   32–3
    leave arrangements   34–6
    leaving the practice   32–4
    legal issues   32–45
    mutual assessment periods   32–3
    progression to parity   32–3
    restrictive covenants   33–4
partnerships   11–45
    banking policy   45
    behaviour   16–23
    Belbin's group roles   17–18
    compatibility issues   5–9
    conflict resolution   18, 19
    culture   13–16
    dynamics   16–23

partnerships (*continued*)
  ethos   13–16
  financial issues   39–45
  formal models   23–31
  groupthink   14, 15–16
  key issues summary   13
  larger practices   18–20
  moral stances   13–15
  number of partners   18–23
  patients list   31
  personal needs   100–4
  premises   36–9
  professional stances   13–15
  religious issues   14, 15
  cf. salaried GPs   48–50
  size   18–23
  small practices   22–3
  small practices linked   20–1
  stereotypes   15–16
  team roles   16–18
paternity leave   35
  general practice   105–6
patient care   3–4
  balance   4–9
patients list, partnerships   31
patients, writing for   85
pay, locums   56, 57, 58, 60
PCTs *see* primary care trusts
personal experiences
  academic general practice   68–9
  salaried GPs   52
  trainers, postgraduate education
    77
personal needs, partnerships   100–4
policies, practice-shaping   23–31
pooling expenses   42–3
pooling income   40–1
postgraduate education   71–9
  course organising   78
  deanery tutors   78–9
  HPE directors   78–9
  structure   72
  trainers   73–7
practice administrators   28–9
practice-based teaching, academic
  general practice   65–8

practice managers   28–9
practice-shaping policies   23–31
premises
  flexibility   37
  leasing   38
  owning   36–7
  partnerships   36–9
  renting   39
primary care trusts (PCTs)
  academic general practice   66
  advantages   93
  characteristics required   92–3
  clinical leads   90–1
  disadvantages   93
  executive committee   90
  expertise areas   92
  opportunities, clinicians'   89–91
  personal experiences   93–5
  points to consider   91–3
  research   68
  salaried GPs   50
  working for   89–95
Prison Medical Service   114–15
private sector GPs   116
professional journals, writing   82–3
professional stances, partnerships
  13–15
progression to parity, Partnership
  Deeds   32–3
The Project Surgery   3
  flexibility   99–103

religious issues
  partnerships   14, 15
  religious observance leave   35
renting premises   39
research
  academic general practice   66–8
  PCTs   68
restrictive covenants, Partnership
  Deeds   33–4

sabbatical leave   35
salaried GPs   31, 47–53
  academic sessions   66
  advantages   48–9

disadvantages   49–50
flexibility   49, 52
GPSRs   51
job applications   51–2
maternity pay   49, 52
options   50–1
cf. partnerships   48–50
PCTs   50
personal experiences   52
sick pay   49, 52
status   49–50
team roles   52
salaried partners   30
secondary type care   109–13
senior partner as executive,
    partnership model   23–4, 27
shares, financial issues   39–40
shark, conflict mode style   19
sick leave   35
sick pay, salaried GPs   49, 52
size, partnerships   18–23
small practices linked, partnerships
    20–1
small practices, partnerships   22–3
sports medicine   115
status, salaried GPs   49–50
stereotypes, partnerships   15–16
study leave   35

tax
    financial issues   39–40
    locums   58, 60
teaching, practice-based, academic
    general practice   65–8
team roles
    partnerships   16–18
    salaried GPs   52
teddy bear, conflict mode style   19
tortoise, conflict mode style   19

trainers, postgraduate education
    73–7
    advantages   73–4
    attributes   76–7
    disadvantages   74–5
    inspection   76
    notes summarisers   76
    pathway   75–6
    personal experiences   77
    VTSs   75
triangle, balance, income/workload/
    patient care   4–9

university-based academic general
    practice   64–5

variety of work   119–20
vocational training schemes (VTSs),
    postgraduate education   75
voluntary sector work   116
VTSs see vocational training schemes

welfare   1–9
women GPs, general practice
    105–7
work flexibility   2–3
workload   1–9
    balance   4–9
writing   81–8
    academic journals   82–3
    advantages   86
    books   84–5
    disadvantages   86–7
    journals   82–3
    for lay press   85
    medical newspapers   83–4
    for patients   85
    professional journals   82–3
    starting   87